PRESCRIPTION TECHNOLOGY

PRESCRIPTION TECHNOLOGY

Opening Physician-Patient Communication Channels

PRANATHI KONDAPANENI, MD, MPH.

Published by Ingenium Books Publishing Inc.
Toronto, Ontario, Canada M6P 1Z2

All rights reserved.
www.ingeniumbooks.com

ISBN:
978-1-989059-10-4 (paperback/softcover)
978-1-989059-11-1 (electronic)
978-1-989059-09-8 (hardcover/hardback)
978-1-989059-12-8 (audiobook)
978-1-989059-16-6 (large print)

Disclaimer

This publication was written by a physician. Material in this book is for education purposes only and is not to be misconstrued as medical advice. The reader has no therapeutic relationship with the physician author. While the publisher and author have made every attempt to verify that the information provided in this book is correct and up to date, the publisher and author assume no responsibility for an error, inaccuracy, or omission.

"Technology is unlocking the innate compassion we have for all our fellow human beings."

—Bill Gates

Contents

Dedication

To my parents, for their loving grace...

To Mahesh, for his practical wisdom...

To Sowmya, for her compassionate faith...

Introduction

WITHOUT WARNING, IT CREEPS into the doctor's office.

Without remorse, it disrupts the doctor's schedule.

Without mercy, it encourages the doctor's frustration.

What is the stealthy troublemaker?

It's the Electronic Medical Record Meltdown!

Many healthcare providers can attest to the pure irritation of an electronic medical record's temper tantrum right in the middle of a busy clinic day. Why do these temper tantrums have to occur when there's a long line of patients in the waiting room?

An electronic medical record meltdown is what happens when the medical frontline reaches its breaking point in dealing with work-hindering technology. For example, in some electronic medical record systems, the number of clicks it takes to schedule a simple follow-up visit for a patient is ridiculous. It can feel as though you're trying to order a nuclear submarine launch. And if you want to order a referral, it's a few more clicks through a different window. In a medical system comprised of physicians and patients already starved for time, these little technological annoyances add up quickly.

In my view, many of these technologies aren't suited to the healthcare provider. Also, physicians are being bombarded with requests and requirements to use multiple technologies at the same time. Medicine is stressful enough without needing to remember multiple logins or user interfaces. The result is money spent on something that physicians won't properly utilize. Why can't technology be built to better support, rather than hurt, the physician-patient relationship?

Technology's penetration of the healthcare sector, compared to other sectors, has been relatively slow due to appropriate concerns regarding protecting patient health and privacy. But given sky-rocketing costs in the sector, incentives to use technology to make healthcare delivery more cost-effective are increasing. In her TED talk, Nadjia Yousif, technology and financial institutions specialist at The Boston Consulting Group, noted that approximately 25 percent of the technology solutions, which companies originally consider adopting, are soon cancelled or sit unused.[1] That's a great deal of money to be left on the table in a cash-strapped health-care system. Therefore, all stakeholders in healthcare should be concerned with implementing technology in a manner that will benefit, rather than hamper, the delivery of healthcare.

How can we implement technology more effectively? It is when we deploy technology through a human lens that we can implement it effectively for both the patient and the physician.

While many healthcare stakeholders are focused on utilizing technology to solve problems, such as optimizing medical supply chains or securing health records against fraud, my interest lies in the more human need for the physician and the patient to connect. Currently, the physician-patient bond is on life support due to ongoing communication barriers within healthcare. In this book, we will explore how technology can break down these barriers and restore the element of human connection to the physician-patient relationship.

My Quest

In the fall of 1997, after reciting the Hippocratic Oath, I was inducted into the world of medicine. This is the line that resonated with me the most:

> *"I will remember that there is art to medicine as well as science and that warmth, sympathy, and understanding may outweigh the surgeon's knife or the chemist's drug."*[2]

As the years passed, my ability to give that warmth, sympathy, and understanding to the patient was severely degraded as a result of an onerous medical system that perversely valued economic incentives over patients' health. To be fair, I didn't know what I was getting into. At the age of sixteen, I was accepted into a combined undergraduate/medical school program. At the age of twenty-four, I had undergraduate degrees in economics and biology, along with a master's in public health and a medical degree.

After medical school, I finished a neurology residency, took a year off to travel, and completed fellowships in epilepsy and sleep medicine. In December 2008, I began what was to become a decade as a private-practice physician. Originally, I had no intention of trying to solve the patient-physician communication barrier. After all, how could I, a simple physician in private practice, take on this whole onerous medical system? I did, however, decide to make a few changes in my own clinical practice.

In January 2015, I embarked on an adventure to learn about communication. I learned everything from observation skills in visual arts to stand-up comedy performances. My quest was to learn as much as I could from artists so I could better communicate with my patients.

During the summer of 2016, my search brought me to the world of design thinking, an iterative process that involves seeking to understand the user, challenge our assumptions, rethink problems, and look for new strategies and solutions. I was part of a diverse team with expertise in design, public health, and user experience, and our task was to design an item to improve the health of a lower-class neighborhood in Washington, DC. We looked at the points where technology and healthcare intersected, and after brainstorming we created a home-health-assistant module for patients: think, Google Home meets home-health aide. These informational sessions re-introduced me to the wonders of technology.

Here I must digress. In my teenage bedroom, the central light fixture was similar to the light fixture in the poker room of *Star Trek: The Next Generation*.[3] As a teenager, I loved this television show—in large part due to a crush on Captain Jean-Luc Picard. However, Captain Jean-Luc aside, the technological possibilities presented in the show seemed endless. The ability to transport matter—as in, a living human being—off a spaceship onto a planet's surface. The glasses that allowed Geordi La Forge, who was blind, to see. The hologram suites that transported people into new worlds. To me, the most fascinating scenes were those in the poker room, where the crew, despite all the technology surrounding them, were more relaxed, more themselves, and more human.

As a child, the intersection of humanity and technology always intrigued me, and during that memorable summer of 2016 I rediscovered that wonderment. While there is quite a bit of literature on how this or that new fancy advancement can deliver better payments or optimize the supply chain, my interest is still in how technology can be used to improve what is so lacking in medicine today: the human connection.

Now, I would not dare to be so bold as to pretend that I'm a technological whiz. I'm the last person to grasp how to work a new remote control. Many experts can eloquently explain the intricacies of technological advancements far better than I can. Yet how many of these technological experts have had to try to communicate complex medical conditions to patients? How many have tried to improve an individual's health by prescribing behavioral changes? How many have done all of this while putting up with a medical system that, in the United States at least, is about as patient-physician friendly as a closed and bolted door?

Many clinical physicians working in academic research on digital medicine do a wonderful job. However, the realities of an average clinical practice are far different from those in academic centers. Given that I'm a regular physician on a mission to improve practical communication in her office, I offer a unique perspective that's often lacking in the medical-technology discussions—that of an ordinary private-practice physician.

This Book's Road Map

The first section of this book explores patient-physician interactions before, during, and after a clinical appointment. In the first chapter of this section, we'll walk through current communication pain-points in a typical patient-physician exchange. In the following two chapters, we'll explore technology's potential to improve the clinical experience. In the fourth chapter, we'll again walk through a typical patient-physician interaction, but this time we'll consider how technology can improve patient-physician communication before, during, and after the clinical appointment.

The second section of this book focuses on what happens in the time between patient-physician clinical appointments.

In the second section, first chapter, we'll discuss how technology can significantly enhance communication to improve patient education. Medicine has three legs: medication, surgery, and lifestyle change. Lifestyle change is an area where technology can make a big difference: it can help to improve patient health outcomes by improving patient education. After all, no matter how effective the patient-physician appointment seems to be, what's the point if the patient doesn't follow the medical treatment plan between appointments? In the next chapter, we'll consider an effective physician-patient communication model in a typical patient-physician scenario. Finally, we'll frame the patient-physician relationship within the larger technological forces shaping our future. It's important for physicians and physician leaders alike to deepen their understanding of technological advancements that will affect healthcare in the future.

I've written this book for physicians and medical leaders, but technology professionals may find this book useful in developing an awareness of how physicians regard technology and of how the growing impact of technology can influence patient care. However, since the book is physician-focused, the emphasis is on the clinical application of general technology concepts.

Technology's Advancement

Technology is changing exponentially. In fact, the technology references in this book may be out of date the day it's published. However, the concepts in this book will live beyond the status of any particular technology. For example, whether you're introduced to medical scanning by a simple x-ray, a CT scan, an MRI, a PET scan, or a functional MRI scan, the concept of imaging a body to help with diagnosis and treatment is still the same. Similarly, no matter what technological medical interventions you're using, the theoretical concepts raised here will still be relevant.

A Thing of Beauty

The physician-patient bond is a very strange creature. As physicians, we may feel as though we've won when our patients' health improves. And we may feel as though we've failed when our patients' health declines.

As I've matured as a physician, I've come to realize that what's most important is not to address symptoms but to heal the whole patient. When a physician truly connects with a patient and can observe how a patient overcomes individual struggles, it's an inspiring experience. If a patient is truly healed and hasn't simply had their symptoms addressed, the physician-patient bond may blossom into an exquisite masterpiece, no matter how long the relationship lasts.

Therefore, to reinstate the beauty of the human connection into the patient-physician bond, let us boldly go where technology and medicine have never gone before.

SECTION ONE:

BEFORE • DURING • AFTER

Chapter 1: Mr. Scotty Spock 1.0

"Most patients enter a doctor's office or hospital as if it were a Mayan temple representing an ancient and mysterious culture with no language in common with the visitor."

—*Tom Brokaw*

DESPITE THE BEST INTENTIONS, both the patient and the physician often feel as though they're speaking different languages during a clinical appointment. Why does this happen? To further our understanding, let's use a typical patient-physician scenario to examine the communication dysfunction that occurs before, during, and after a clinical office visit. Imagine that this appointment is set during 2018 in the United States.

Before the Office Visit: Friday, 4:30 P.M.

Dr. Dianna Crusher:

As raindrops dribble down the office window, Dr. Crusher bends over her computer, her thoughts awash in frustration. She thinks:

One last patient to go. I wish I was done after that! But my inbox is stuffed with messages. I still have to dictate all my patient notes. The cherry on top is that lovely administration-

required quality-review training. I didn't go to med school to figure out if I'm meeting government regulations. You would think that someone else should be doing that. But no, the doctor has to treat the patients, keep track of regulations, do the billing, and keep all the staff happy. By the time I'm done with all this, it's going to be well past seven o'clock. Oh crap, I forgot to call the babysitter to stay late! She's going to charge me an arm and a leg. Damn it! The kids are going to be so pissed. I promised them I'd be home for dinner. Lovely start to the weekend. Just lovely!

As Dr. Crusher is rubbing her eyelids, a notification pops up on her computer. Her last patient has checked in for his appointment. She glances through his online chart.

Hmm. I first saw Mr. Scotty Spock four months ago. I don't really remember him. Of course, given that I have 1500 patients in my practice, it's impossible for me to remember someone I've seen only once. Looks like he's here for his first follow-up: a blood-pressure check. He was supposed to be on a diet-and-exercise-modification program. It seems his weight is creeping up. We need to talk about weight-loss clinics or surgery or medication options. How am I supposed to cover everything in fifteen minutes?

Mr. Scotty Spock:

As raindrops drip down the waiting-room window, Scotty shifts restlessly in his chair and clenches his hands, wishing he didn't have to be here.

What a day to come clear across town in rush-hour traffic. And, of course, the doctor is running late. Instead of letting me leave early, my boss made me use up my last vacation day for this bloody appointment. He's a lousy oaf! I still had to go into the office to finish up my project this morning. It's not like I had much of a choice about the appointment scheduling. This doctor is like every other doctor. Booked out! If I hadn't kept this appointment, I would have had to wait another two months. This doctor had better spend some real time with me!

Mr. Scotty Spock's name is called. With a hunched back and thoughts mirroring his posture, he walks toward the doctor's examination room.

Three months. Three long months since I had a good night's sleep. What I really need is rest. But will the doctor help me with that? No, she'll probably just tell me again to eat better and get more exercise. Yeah, right. How can I do that when I'm working eighty hours a week and can still hardly get by? I've got to work two jobs or no house payment. And the kids. I have to take care of the kids! I used to make better money. But just as I turned sixty, the pink slip was in my mailbox. I've got to work where I can. Is seeing this doctor even worth it? On top of this fifty-dollar co-pay, there's the cost of gas to get over here, wasting my last vacation day, and not even getting paid for the work I had to do this morning. This day has been a total loss!

Discussion

Consider the mindsets of the doctor and the patient before the appointment. Both are human, their thoughts and emotions framing the day's events.

Dr. Crusher seems burdened, even overwhelmed, by the pile of unfinished tasks not directly related to patient care: a full email inbox, administrative work, charting patient notes. (Patients and others outside the healthcare system tend not to know about the time and energy physicians spend on non-clinical tasks.) She has to manage multilayered clinical tasks, including reviewing each patient's chart before the visit. With a caseload of 1500 patients, it's difficult—even impossible—to remember the clinical details of each of them. Dr. Crusher also worries about caring for her children, a reminder that physicians, too, have loved ones and personal lives, and those needs can overflow into clinical time. Finally, Dr. Crusher wants to spend more time with her patients instead of performing non-patient related tasks. This is, after all, why she went to medical school.

Scotty is also frustrated, but for different reasons. He seems to resent using a vacation day to see the doctor—a relatively common situation. Scotty tallies up the occupational costs, transportation costs, personal costs, and insurance costs for this appointment. In addition, Scotty has to worry about co-pays, varying deductibles, and other healthcare costs. Moreover, his personal and family stresses increase his general anxiety. Finally, he's taken notice that the physician is already late for the appointment. Will she give him the time he needs?

Already we see that the physician and the patient have different agendas for the visit. The patient expects the doctor to address his sleep issues. But the doctor wants to address the patient's weight control. Both are additionally stressed out by workload and personal worries. Thus, their priorities in terms of health concerns aren't the same. Before the patient even steps inside the doctor's office, he's been set up for a very poor visit, indeed!

During the Office Visit: Friday, 4:55 P.M.

Dr. Dianna Crusher:
Tired of counseling the patient on weight loss, Dr. Crusher repeatedly taps on her computer keyboard. The screen is frozen.

Why doesn't he listen? Doesn't he get it? If he keeps on this trajectory—ten pounds every few months—by the end of the year, he could weigh forty to fifty more pounds. This is really important. Weight gain leads to increased blood pressure and increased risk of diabetes. He needs to be careful. But does he care? Apparently not! Hmmm. This despicable electronic medical record is giving me another screen to click through. How many clicks do I have to make to get a referral for a weight-loss clinic? And, man, I'm hungry! The last time I ate was at breakfast. Of course, with the constant phone calls, forget lunch!

Finally, the computer screen moves, and the weight-loss referral prints. Dr. Crusher pulls it from the printer and hands it to the patient, who looks totally miffed.

It's not my fault, buddy, that you put on ten pounds. I'm sorry, too, that you're not sleeping right, but proper diet and exercise would help. If you have a sugary diet and don't move all day, you're not going to sleep well. But do you ever listen to me? No! The higher your weight gets, the harder it will be to lose it. Hmmmm. I still haven't called the babysitter to ask her to stay late!

Mr. Scotty Spock:
Scotty grabs the referral angrily.

Why is she not listening to me? I'm not sleeping, lady! I know my stupid weight is a problem. But how am I supposed to get to the gym or shop and make the kind of food you want me to eat if I only have two or three hours of sleep a night? I don't want this stupid referral to a weight-loss clinic. Like it's going to do any good? Oh yippee-do-da-day!

A weight loss-clinic with a ton more appointments, and for sure a bunch of co-pays with money I don't have. Does this doctor think I'm made of gold?

Scotty sighs as Dr. Crusher turns her back to him—her computer has started beeping again.

That darned computer is getting more attention than me. She doesn't even look me in the eye. She keeps clicking and staring into that screen. You'd think with her fancy degree and fancy paycheck, she could get a computer that wouldn't keep chirping. Can't you shut it up? Oh no, now my phone's going off. And yikes, at this rate, I'm going to be seriously late getting home for dinner. I forgot to tell the kids to order pizza before I got there. Well, none of us are starving. Seriously, why, why, why doesn't the doctor ever listen to me? I need help with my sleep, lady!

Discussion

Neither party is having a good office visit.

The physician is frustrated that the patient doesn't appear to be listening to her regarding his weight. The patient is frustrated that the physician doesn't appear to be listening to him regarding his need to sleep. It's not uncommon for doctors and patients to have different agendas during clinical appointments, and when this happens, both parties may become frustrated and feel unheard.

Additionally, many issues—such as every frustrating and time-consuming keyboard click that comes with the electronic medical records—can exacerbate the interaction and make the time-limited encounter less patient-focused. Finally, both parties are human, and outside stressors such as family needs can easily ratchet up the resentment growing from unmet agendas and computer-induced disconnection.

After the Office Visit: Friday, 5:30 P.M.

Dr. Dianna Crusher:
   As rain thrashes against her office window, Dr. Crusher yawns and stares aimlessly into the computer screen.

> *An inbox full of messages, patient notes to dictate, and that damn quality review for the administration! I'll be here for hours. Why did Mr. Spock show up for his appointment today? He didn't listen to one thing I had to say! Last time, I gave him a bunch of websites so he could read up on weight loss. Did he read any of them? No! I told him how to cook at home, use portion control, and increase his daily activity to lose weight. Did he remember any of it? No!*

She reaches in the drawer for her phone to call the babysitter. Seeing the time, she sighs.

> *Now, I have to spend another fifteen minutes writing the note about his visit. If only I could actually spend more time with patients instead of spending all this time on notes, messages, and so much administration, even my worst days would be more tolerable.*

Mr. Scotty Spock:
   As the rain pours on his car window, Mr. Spock yawns and tosses his weight-loss referral on the passenger seat.

> *What a waste of my time! The doctor was more interested in her computer than in me! How am I supposed to remember*

all the stuff she tells me at every visit? And those websites she sends me to are useless, either written in medical speak or just plain boring. I don't have time to get a degree in weight loss. I've got a life to live.

He groans as he checks his phone for the traffic report.

Oh, no, an accident on the highway! I'm going to be stuck in traffic for at least an hour. And for what? She was no help at all for my sleep. I don't want another referral. I want real help! I wish I could get my money back for today's visit. And reimbursed for my time and lost vacation day. What do these doctors think, that we have endless time and money? Forget this weight-loss clinic! I'm done seeing doctors. I'm done wasting my time on visits that don't help me!

Discussion

Both parties left the appointment quite unhappy.

The physician was not only overloaded with nonmedical tasks but also frustrated that the patient hadn't followed through with her medical advice from the last visit. She also resented that she wasn't properly compensated for her professional time, as she spent so much unpaid time on tasks not directly related to patient care.

The patient was aware of how difficult it would be to follow the medical advice, in terms of reading, treatment plans, and other appointments. With so much going on in his life, how can he complete all the required tasks? He worried about the unaffordable costs which would result if he followed through with the weight lost referral.

Neither felt listened to during the appointment, and both were stressed out by family needs and schedules. The final result was poor for both the burned-out physician and the noncompliant patient.

The Communication Conundrum

The above example can be summed up in two words: poor communication.

What does "communication" really mean? On a basic level, communication is the act of transmitting ideas, thoughts, or emotions. Communication occurs in many ways: spoken words, nonverbal gestures, signs, and symbols. We also use various channels, or media, to communicate messages. Examples of media include newspapers, songs, television, or virtual reality experiences.

In addition, there are many levels of communication.[4] I'm going to talk about five:

1. Societal communication. On a basic level, societal communication, e.g., news channels on TV, is aimed at a mass audience.
2. Institutional communication, e.g., an office memo circulating through a company's email chain, is aimed at large institutions.
3. Group communication, e.g., staff updates regarding personnel changes.
4. Interpersonal communication, e.g., two friends meeting for coffee, exists between two or more people.
5. Finally, intrapersonal communication includes communication one has with him/herself.

In our scenario, communication breakdowns occurred on all these levels.

From a societal communication standpoint, the patient-physician relationship is held to an unrealistic expectation. In the

Saturday Evening Post on April 12, 1947, there was an illustration by Norman Rockwell entitled *Country Doctor.*[5] In this idealized picture, a genial-looking physician is sitting down with a young family. The physician and the family are facing each other and making eye contact, and everyone seems comfortable. No one looks rushed. Both sides seem ripe for a substantive discussion. This is the type of interaction that both patients and physicians yearn for. However, the reality is radically different. The fifteen-minute-appointment norm for returning patients combined with alienation caused by the computer being placed between the patient and the physician means we're a long way off from what Norman Rockwell painted nearly seventy years ago.

In terms of institutional communication, the patient-physician relationship cannot get a break. The messages the patient received from his work and his insurance didn't help the situation. In our scenario, the patient had to take a vacation day to keep his appointment. While this may not be the case in all workplaces, it's not uncommon for patients to ask me to reschedule appointments because they can't get time off work. They also reschedule because they have to attend to family issues or cannot get transportation. The institutions surrounding the patient (e.g., workplace, childcare facility) send direct or indirect messages that the patient's health isn't important. The most direct of these messages often comes from the health insurance companies—at least within the United States in 2018. When money is at the core of healthcare, a medical visit can feel transactional. I believe it should feel experiential instead.

In our scenario, Dr. Crusher had much more work to do after Scotty's visit: check email, dictate patient notes, and finish administrative assessments. While some of these tasks are important, the healthcare system is not set up to optimize physicians' time. Instead of helping patients, physicians waste their time on needless tasks that sap their energy and drain their resources.

Healthcare systems send the message to physicians that time for patients is not that important. This is a reality of everyday clinical practice.

From a group communication standpoint, the patient-physician relationship is often strained by the groups to which the parties belong to outside the patient-physician relationship. In our scenario, both the physician and the patient were worried about their children. The physician forgot to call the babysitter to ask her to stay late. The patient forgot to tell his kids to order dinner because he was going to be late. Each party's failure to communicate properly with their families burdened both parties and strained the visit even more.

On an interpersonal level, additional lapses in communications occurred. It's important to note that neither felt heard. The patient clearly believed his major issue was lack of sleep. The physician's main concern was the patient's weight gain. Both of these issues were important. However, their differing priorities and inability to truly listen to each other compounded the miscommunication. The physician was frustrated because the patient failed to follow the plan of care and hadn't even looked at the websites she'd suggested. Yet these avenues of information weren't beneficial to the patient. So, on top of miscommunication, we have a mismatch in priorities and ineffective education after the clinical visit. Moreover, the patient was frustrated by the physician's lack of eye contact. The physician was frustrated by the computer itself. This lack of proper nonverbal connection significantly worsened the dynamic.

Finally, both the patient and physician suffered in terms of their intrapersonal relationship. The patient resented not only that his major issue, poor sleep, was never addressed but also that he suffered financial costs: loss of pay for working the morning, loss of a vacation day, loss of the co-pay and loss of the transportation costs. The physician resented the wasted time she could have spent eating lunch, reading emails, and dictating notes. These differing but important resentments further soured their relationship.

The Resulting Communication Breakdown

The purpose of dissecting communications theory is to illustrate the complex ways in which communication broke down on multiple levels in our clinical scenario. What's truly sad is how quite common this scenario is in contemporary healthcare.

If one were to examine more patient-physician examples, additional variations of communication breakdowns would undoubtedly emerge. It's critical to understand the communication conundrum from the point of view of both physicians and patients. When communications go wrong, patients often become less invested in their health and less compliant with physicians' treatment plans. Poorer health outcomes for the patient are often the result.

When communication breaks down, physicians often feel like banging their heads against a wall. Are we wasting time talking to patients when they don't follow through on our best professional advice? Improving the health of our patients is a main source of job satisfaction for us. While I don't deny that some physicians may be mercenary by nature, I still believe most went to medical school to help their patients. If becoming a doctor were only a matter of making money, medicine might not be such a vocational bargain, given the many years spent in training. Besides, the stress that results from these communication breakdowns often contributes to physician burnout and, ultimately, zombie physicians who feel disenfranchised and disenchanted.

What can we do about this communication breakdown?

Employ technology.

By learning to let technology help us rather than hinder us, I believe we can mend the physician-patient communication illness and finally allow the physician and patient to speak the same language in the clinical office. However, before we can heal this relationship, we need to understand the technology that will make a huge difference in medicine's future.

Chapter 2: The Promise of Technology

> *"Any sufficiently advanced technology is indistinguishable from magic."*
> —Arthur C. Clarke

TECHNOLOGY HAS THE POWER to accomplish what we once thought was only possible in the realm of magic.

Black Panther is a 2018 film set in the fictional African country of Wakanda. Wakanda appears to the outside world to be a poor country with few resources. Yet, hidden within the mountains and waterfalls is a technological wonderland that's far ahead of the rest of the planet. A CIA agent riddled with bullets during a car chase is healed overnight by a Wakanda resident and is up and walking around the very next day. When the agent asks if he's been healed by magic, he's told instead it was technology.[6]

As technology speeds ahead, what was once thought to be in the realm of magic is now becoming an everyday reality. Within medicine, one such technological reality gaining traction is virtual communication. When I was in medical school, the thought of seeing and talking to a person via computer screen wasn't even discussed. In the last few years, the ability to see your physician on-line has come into vogue, becoming the preferred method of interaction for some patients.

Call me old-fashioned, but there's something to be said for in-person encounters. While I love how long-distance encounters using FaceTime on the computer allow me to talk more often to loved ones who are a world away, certain things can't be replicated through a virtual meeting—the nuance of an expression, the light in someone's eyes, the warmth of a touch. Nothing can replace an actual meeting with someone I care about personally.

However, virtual appointments with a physician will benefit the majority of patients. This is especially true given the shortage of healthcare providers in many areas and the difficulty many patients have traveling to and attending appointments in person.

Whether the future clinical visit is in-person or virtual, the physician will have many new tools with which to help their patients. Although it's impossible to predict all the technologies that will shape the future of healthcare, remote-monitoring and voice-first are two such technological tools which I believe will play an important role in improving communication between physicians and patients.

Remote Monitoring

White coat hypertension is a common healthcare phenomenon: a patient's blood pressure can increase as a result of anxiety caused by merely being in a doctor's office. If medical decisions regarding lifestyle modifications and medications are made based on an inaccurate blood-pressure reading, the implications can be serious. Nowadays, however, patients are able to take their blood pressure at home with low-cost monitors. Thus, using remote monitoring, physicians can spot a valid trend, rather than basing a medical decision on one invalid number. Due to this technological advance, the ability to remotely monitor medical parameters (such as diastolic pressure, systolic pressure, pulse, oxygen saturation levels, etcetera) will explode in the coming years.

The Internet of Things

Fast forward a few years into the future. Imagine this:

You're in your kitchen, walking by Frasier the Fridge. Frasier lets you know that you're low on milk and apples and asks if you want to order some. You say yes. A few hours later, the groceries are delivered. Then you decide that a sandwich would be great with that apple. So, you ask Tony the Toaster to toast up some bread. Tony asks how toasty you'd like it. You say medium would be great. The toast is done to your exact specifications. Then you ask Mindy the Microwave to warm up some soup to go along with that sandwich. Mindy asks how hot you want the soup. You tell her, and the soup is warmed to, you guessed it, your exact specifications. Now you can sit down for a good dinner while watching your favorite television show on Tessa the Table.

Does the scenario sound a little crazy? Well, it may be a reality sooner than you think due to a technological phenomenon called the Internet of Things. The idea is that everyday physical objects, such as tables, fridges, and vehicles, will be embedded with computing devices connected to the internet, so they'll have the ability to send and share information. Already we're starting to see this in action. For example, with Nest smart home devices, a customer can monitor and adjust various thermostats by using a phone app.[7]

From a medical standpoint, computing devices embedded in things such as a fridge or a heating system could give valuable clues as to a patient's environment. For example, does the patient get colds more so during seasonal changes or just during cold weather? Data embedded in physical objects will give the clinician a wealth of information as to which clinical parameters can be correlated.

On a minor scale, I've already seen this with sleep patients. A CPAP machine is commonly used to treat a condition called sleep apnea. It enables a patient to breathe at night by pumping pressurized air into the airway so that the muscles don't collapse onto the throat. Sensors embedded in CPAP machines monitor a patient's usage. These sensors are connected to the internet and wirelessly upload clinical information. If this data indicates a patient isn't doing well, the machine's pressure parameters can be changed remotely.

The future medical possibilities of this technology are exciting.

What if breathing data from a CPAP machine could be paired with humidification figures from the home thermostat? Often in sleep apnea treatment, CPAP tubing can be hampered by differences in the humidity of the air in the tubing and the humidity of the surrounding air.

Another application could use data on television usage. Is the patient's decreased CPAP usage due to difficulty tolerating the machine, or is the problem that the patient stayed up late watching a basketball game? When data collection can be correlated in an appropriate manner, the clinical possibilities are endless.

Portable Monitoring

While monitoring embedded in stationary physical objects is a particularly exciting possibility, already there's an increase in the use of portable monitoring. For example, some Apple Watch models can now monitor EKGs as a screening tool for cardiac patients.[8] This ability to monitor can extend beyond electronic devices. Tattoos are currently being developed for the purpose of medical monitoring. For example, researchers at Harvard and the Massachusetts Institute of Technology have developed a tattoo that can measure the concentration of glucose, sodium, and pH in the interstitial fluid of the skin. An application would let a specifically tattooed individual know when it was time to drink water during exercise. Meantime, researchers at the University of California San Diego have developed a temporary tattoo to monitor people who have diabetes. No pinpricks would definitely increase compliance in diabetic monitoring![9]

Remote monitoring can also play a vital role in returning a patient to a state of functionality. For example, Dynamic Body Technology is a South African company which is developing a system to track movement in real time using Bluetooth sensors. The data can be monitored remotely by a medical professional. As a result, the medical professional can set new goals for the patient to achieve between medical visits and thus, move a patient more quickly to a place of functionality. In addition, such data can give the medical professional objective data regarding a patient's functionality. For example, some patients may feel better even though their range of motion hasn't gotten better after surgery. On the other hand, some patients may not feel better even though their range of motion has significantly improved. The real-time objective data on the range of motion can be correlated with a patient's subjective concerns to determine an appropriate next step.[10]

Limitations of Remote Monitoring

While it's wonderful to be able to collect this medical data, it's also important to determine what data is clinically significant and what data is not. Physicians have limited amounts of time. Therefore, technology needs to play a large role in sorting through data supplied by remote monitoring and presenting what is clinically significant. If a physician has questions about a reading—perhaps they want to know the time of the reading—then more specific data can be accessed when required.

In addition, too much focus on the mounds of data can make a patient lose sight of the bigger picture and even become obsessed with particular numbers. For example, among my insomniacs, I don't recommend tracking sleep with an electronic device. I find that certain insomniacs become so obsessed with their sleep numbers—tracking them not just day to day but hour to hour—that they develop anxiety over sleep itself. This anxiety in turn may negatively affect their ability to fall and stay asleep, which may negatively affect their metrics, which may negatively affect the anxiety—so goes the vicious cycle. In essence, remote monitoring presents a lot of additional medical information which is wonderful when used correctly.

Voice First

Whether you call your electronic helper Alexa, Cortana, Google, Siri, or some other name, you're likely accustomed to activating your electronic devices by voice. In the future, the importance of voice will only grow—and this will have large ramifications for the medical community.

Voice Search

As a child, I would pore over books under my pillow with a little light. A good story would keep me up all night, even if it was time to go to sleep. Fast-forward to 2018; the good story that keeps me up all night is now delivered as an audiobook. Audio media's popularity is rising fast and furiously.

In audio consumption, we need to better develop the algorithms for voice search. In the future, instead of typing search terms into Google to find the nearest urgent care center which could bandage a bad cut, patients of the future will be asking Siri how to bandage up a cut themselves. Voice search is already here. But the populations I'm most eager to see take advantage of voice search are the elderly and the disabled. With voice search, an elderly woman who's immobile can call her home-health aide robot to her side. Or a man who's blind can order medications online. We just need to train all patients how to use it to their advantage.

Moreover, the work burden of medical professionals will be lessened by voice commands. Instead of having to review different screens or click through multiple pages, they can save valuable time by using voice commands to pull up patient information quickly and efficiently.

Electronic Medical Record 2.0

The electronic medical record is another area of great potential within this voice revolution. One of the greatest banes of a physician's existence is the need to write medical notes. Ideally, a medical note would be written right after a patient visit, so that the physician can recall as much detail as possible. In reality, these notes are often finished at the end of the day. Actually, considering a typical day in a clinical office—with appointments interrupted by phone calls, patients delayed due to traffic, and computer glitches—it's a wonder that some physicians get to eat during the day, never mind finish up all the notes. In addition, during the visit itself, physicians often try to make notes on a computer to help them construct an accurate medical note after the visit. But this precludes meaningful eye contact between patient and physician and may also cause the doctor to miss vital nonverbal cues from the patient.

Another ongoing patient issue which virtual visits could address is the difficulty of fully understanding all that's being said by a patient who isn't a native speaker of the physician's language. When a patient is from Guatemala and the doctor from the Philippines, both may be speaking English, but details may be lost in translation. Important details—some nonverbal, others cultural, and still other details like the quality of an abdominal pain—can help the physician with diagnosis but may be left out or misstated by an interpreter.

All of these problems can be addressed by technology. In early 2018, I watched a Microsoft conference presentation demonstrating a virtual office meeting. As the meeting unfolded, the computer automatically took notes, made up an action plan, and translated what office members located in other countries contributed to the meeting. The computer was even able to post images of the building plans under consideration.[11]

Let's transfer the above scenario to a medical office setting. A patient is now able to talk directly to the physician on the computer screen. Any language difference is automatically translated. The computer takes notes as the patient and physician talk. The medical note is generated while the visit is happening. Based on the visit, a plan of action written in easy-to-understand language is generated and given to the patient. The next appointment and referrals are generated as well, based on the conversation during the visit. In addition, the physician can pull up an image of the patient's chest, for example, and share it with the patient, in a sort of 3-D projection, so the patient can see what's going on in their body.

Wouldn't all that be wonderful?

The good news is that we're already starting to go in that direction. Currently Google is working with physicians at Stanford to develop a system in which notes are automatically written as the visit unfolds in real time, so that the physician doesn't have to dictate or type the note later. Dr. Steven Lin, the Stanford physician spearheading the research with Google, told CNBC that the speech recognition systems need to accurately "listen in" to a patient visit and simultaneously parse out the relevant information into a useful narrative.[12]

This type of electronic medical record system has the potential to decrease errors in medical notes substantially. Often, physicians have so many notes to complete that, working at top speed, errors in spelling and wording—although hopefully not in diagnoses or treatment plans—can creep into notes. In the past, when notes were dictated to an assistant instead of a machine, a second set of eyes would often correct these mistakes. But to decrease costs, many physicians had to start typing their own notes directly or dictating them into a transcribing machine. In the future, virtual clinical visits will free the physician to spend more time with the patient. What an advance for the physician: better patient care and less time searching for typos in notes.

I remember hearing, back in med school, about what was to come someday with this magical new technology. Now, it's almost here!

Chapter 3: The Promise of Artificial Intelligence

"I believe this artificial intelligence is going to be our partner. If we misuse it, it will be a risk. If we use it right, it can be our partner."

—Masayoshi Son

WHILE THE PROMISE OF remote-monitoring and voice-first technology are set to play an important role in healthcare, the major game-changer for the future of patient-physician communication is artificial intelligence, or AI.

In the Iron Man movies, Tony Stark is a superhero who combines his robotic ingenuity with human intelligence. Yet, Tony Stark's conquests would not be accomplished without Jarvis, his supercharged AI sidekick.[13] We may not all be superheroes, but our definition of medicine, as we know it, will be forever changed by the partnership of AI and medicine.

Origins of Artificial Intelligence

In his book on AI, Dr. Kai-Fu Lee discusses its origins. In the mid-1950s, the mission to replicate human intelligence broke into two camps. The first was a rules-based approach which tried to teach a computer to think with logic and rules. The second was a neural-networks approach, a computer system based on the human brain and the nervous system, which tried to replicate the human brain.[14]

With a rules-based approach, you would tell the computer the rules to follow in identifying a dog. For example, a dog walks on four legs and barks. With the neural-networks approach, you would feed the network a lot of information, including pictures of dogs and pictures without dogs. Then, the neural networks would learn to identify patterns in the data that would allow the computer to identify a dog.

In the early 2000s, AI gained traction due to two major factors—the internet and computing speed. The vast expanses of the internet gave the neural networks an unmatched reservoir of data from which they could learn, and increased computing power became the fuel that neural networks needed to learn at an accelerated pace. How much computing power? Dr. Kai-Fu Lee estimates a contemporary smartphone has more computing power than the computer NASA used to send Neil Armstrong to the moon. By 2012, a researcher named Jeffrey Hinton and his team were using neural networks to beat their competitors at a world-wide computer contest. After this competition, awareness of AI's potential grew from limited academic circles to the wider world stage.[15]

Definitions of Artificial Intelligence

The terms "artificial intelligence," "deep learning," "machine learning," and "neural networks" are often used interchangeably, but each is a bit different. If you were to imagine circles of meaning within each other, artificial intelligence would be the outermost circle. Essentially, AI is the ability of machines to demonstrate human behavior.

AI can be narrow or general. Most people talk about narrow AI, which optimizes one specific outcome. For example, after feeding a computer program a large amount of data regarding what good credit looks like, a narrow AI program can identify good candidates for home loans. But general AI in its broadest sense encompasses the ideal of replicating the full range of human intelligence. In the near future, however, we're more likely to see a human enhanced by AI than general AI.

"Machine learning" is an umbrella term that refers to the specific route by which AI is achieved, such as the technique we've been discussing in which machines are fed large amounts of data. The machines learn from the data and then predict an outcome based on the data.

Deep learning is a subset of machine learning. It's a specific methodology using neural networks to perform machine learning. A neural network is a computer system which is modeled on the human brain and the nervous system. It attempts to replicate the functions of the human brain.

Artificial Intelligence in the Real World

I welcome Netflix notifications suggesting a new show for me to enjoy. Sometimes the suggestions are great finds, and sometimes they're not to my taste. When I like a suggestion, I add it to my "to-watch" list or watch it and rate it positively. The more feedback I give the algorithm, the more Netflix can learn my preferences and make better suggestions based on my feedback. This process of doing, learning, redoing, and relearning is at the heart of the concept that underlies AI.

Internet Artificial Intelligence

Dr. Kai-Fu Lee describes the four waves of AI that appear at different times in the application of AI.[16]

The first wave is internet AI, and it first occurred in 1998. The more data a program has, the better the outcome it can produce. Therefore, most of the current giants of AI are internet companies. An example of internet AI is Google's use of previous search data to optimize ads.

Business Artificial Intelligence

The second wave of AI is business AI, and it began in 2004. In this wave, corporations (such as banks, insurance agencies, or hospitals), which have historically stored data for legal or other reasons, buy AI from a supplier. Then the stored data and the AI are used in combination to improve the performance of a business function. For example, a bank can use stored data on previous customers to develop an algorithm to pick better loan candidates.

Perception Artificial Intelligence

The third wave is perception AI, and it first came about in 2011. The algorithm digitizes the surrounding physical world and stores information that was previously considered transient, such as images and sound. For example, Amazon Go stores serve customers based on facial recognition.[17] Data is generated by sensing sight, sound, heat, etc. It functions like added ears and eyes for the computer algorithm. Perception AI appears particularly useful in terms of remote monitoring for patients. For example, it could help monitor an elderly patient who's at risk of falling, or a patient with disabilities who may have trouble swallowing medications.

Autonomous Artificial Intelligence

The fourth wave is autonomous AI, and it started in 2015. If wave three added eyes and ears, wave four added hands and legs.

Fused with a robotic element, autonomous AI has mechanical energy and mechanical dexterity. An example of the fourth wave is self-driving cars, such as those developed by Waymo. At first, the company made the cars drive millions of miles to feed the algorithm data on how to drive. The cars developed a large-enough data set that they now simulate driving conditions to self-improve the algorithm.[18]

Artificial Intelligence Applied to Medicine

Moorfields Eye Hospital is a well-regarded ophthalmology institution in London. In 2016, it partnered with DeepMind, an AI company acquired by Google in 2014. DeepMind published research in July 2018 based on its collaboration with Moorfields. This research showed how AI technology was able to detect eye conditions in a few seconds, indicating that AI could prioritize patients who need urgent care.[19] An AI triage system which matches the accuracy of trained human physicians could revolutionize the practice of medicine.

This represents only a sliver of AI's potential power to revolutionize medicine. Another important area of application would be patient-information gathering. Chris Waugh, chief innovation officer at Sutter Health, discussed in the *Creative Confidence Series* podcast how using AI could improve a patient's writing of a living will.[20] He proposed using AI to analyze how questions are asked (such as the order of questions), so that more patients are encouraged to write a living will. Current medical wisdom states that clarity in end-of-life instructions and expectations in a living will can alleviate suffering for both families and patients.

Finally, AI has the potential to alleviate some common problems for physicians regarding electronic communication, such as inboxes saturated with messages and mounds of records to review. AI can learn a physician's preferences and then prioritize important emails. It can also learn how to review medical data and sort out what's important to the physician.

For example, toe-bunion removal is not a high priority for a sleep physician like me, unless something such as resulting pain from the procedure is affecting the patient's ability to sleep. In such a clinical case, looking at the patient's foot would be more beneficial than looking at the computer screen. I wish some administrators understood this basic concept!

The Medical "Jarvis"

In the medical world of the future, wouldn't it be wonderful to have an AI system to augment—not replace—the physician, just like the Jarvis in the Iron Man movies? While there is already talk of some medical specialities, such as radiology, going by the wayside due to AI, specialties which require a high degree of human touch will most likely remain.

For AI to benefit the healthcare provider, new pathways need to be tested in real time and possibly recalibrated based on user feedback. This process is important to ensure the technology is useful and not a hindrance. If AI is tested and recalibrated correctly, we physicians can look forward to using our own "Medical Jarvis"—a valuable weapon in our medical arsenal to help treat the patient.

Chapter 4: Mr. Scotty Spock 2.0

"The good physician treats the disease. The great physician treats the patient who has the disease."

—William Osler

EVEN THOUGH A PATIENT may come to a physician with a specific medical disease, the underlying issues are often more than just a medical condition. The medical ideal is to treat the whole patient, not just the disease state. With the help of technology, this ideal can be achieved.

In Chapter 1, we looked at an office visit which left both the patient and the physician unsatisfied.

Let's reconsider this visit, but this time we'll set it in 2030 and use some of the new technologies I've described.

Before the Visit: Friday, 4:25 P.M.

Mr. Scotty Spock:

Scotty closes the door to his home office and sits down at his desk. On his computer, he's connected to the patient portal, which prompts him to enter the major concern he wants addressed during this visit. He types in, "I'm having difficulty sleeping because of the noises outside my house." After a message pops up to let him know the doctor will be with him shortly, the patient portal asks th is favorite music is. Scotty enters "Klingon Chamber Music."

Dr. Dianna Crusher:

Dr. Crusher's large wall-mounted monitor flickers and sings out, "4:30 p.m. patient." She glances up at Mr. Scotty Spock's photograph and chart summary. She says aloud, "*Last set of home vitals, please,*" and then studies the information which appears on the screen. She enters the major issue she wants addressed during this visit: Weight gain. She's also able to see that the patient's major issue is not sleeping well, and she's able to accesses relevant information regarding his clinical sleep history. Before she connects with Scotty, Dr. Crusher continues to study his data, including new stats supplied by his home monitoring. Based on the data, she can assess that his sleep is restless, and his weight has gone up. Also, his home audio system indicates a nighttime increase in disruptive bedroom noise.

As she waits to be connected to the patient via videoconferencing, her mind ponders her previous professional life.

> *My inbox is empty. I have no notes to do. And I love how the computer keeps track of admin stuff! I used to hate doing those stupid administrative, quality-review assessments.*

Mr. Scotty Spock:

As he happily reclines in his brand-new comfy office chair, Scotty reads about his upcoming appointment. His half-hour appointment will be broken down as follows: five minutes for saying hello, ten minutes for his sleeping complaints, and fifteen minutes for the rest of his interactions with the doctor. He smiles as the patient portal notifies him that the doctor has already reviewed his sleep-history stats.

During the Visit: Friday, 4:30 P.M. to 5:00 P.M.

Dr. Dianna Crusher:

When the visit commences, she discusses basic sleep-hygiene techniques with Scotty and prescribes specific earplugs. She's happy to address his concern about not sleeping and is able to explain how weight gain can be connected to his inability to get a good night's sleep. She prescribes a set of nutrition plans, which she sends electronically to his home health-aide robot, Rhonda. In addition, Dr. Crusher talks to Mr. Spock about exercise. Since he really likes playing with his kids, she suggests a series of games they can all play together so he can both exercise and spend quality time with his children. She devotes the visit's final five minutes to answering the patient's questions. They agree to schedule an appointment in three months, which the patient portal automatically schedules. She thinks:

Wow, I think he finally understands why it's important to not gain weight and how weight gain can worsen his sleep. I love the fact that we were able to come up with an exercise program which will allow him to spend time with his kids. This way, he's more likely to stick to it. And with Rhonda's help, he should be able to eat well enough to control his weight. All in all, I love how I was able to help the patient by our coming up with a game plan together. He actually listened to what I had to say!

After the Visit: Friday, 5:00 P.M.

Mr. Scotty Spock:

The patient portal, before closing, asks him if he's happy with the visit and ready to pay the twenty-five-dollar co-pay. He says yes, and immediately the payment is electronically processed. His smartphone inbox receives details regarding his exercise and nutrition, as well as specifics on which earplugs to buy. His home entertainment system has already been loaded with games he can play with his children. He decides to play the bowling game with them for an hour. Then, at dinner, he enjoys a healthy dinner Rhonda has prepared according to the doctor's recommendations. His son tells him about a basketball game which will conflict with his next doctor's appointment. After dinner, he has the patient portal change the appointment. Later in the evening, after his shower, he inserts the earplugs the pharmacy delivered according to the doctor's prescription. He thinks:

> *Great, these earplugs are nice and soft and fit right into my ear. They actually block the noise! So much better than regular earplugs! And I can't believe that dinner was healthy. It was really delicious. Also, the exercise wore me out. The best part was playing with the kids. It really helped me de-stress. I think I'm going to have a beautiful night's sleep!*

Dr. Dianna Crusher:

After the visit is finished, she hears a welcome message from her computer: "Done for the day, Dr. Crusher." The computer has already filed the medical note, her inbox is empty, and she has no administrative work. In addition, the computer automatically took care of the billing for the visit. She can be home soon.

> *Done for the day! I love the fact that all I have to do is concentrate on treating the patient. Once I'm home, I can concentrate on just being with my family. This weekend, I'm going to take the kids to visit their grandparents. Maybe while we're there, we can put together that family photo book we've been talking about for so long. This weekend is going*

to be lovely. Then, come Monday morning, I'll be refreshed, rejuvenated, and ready to get my patients healthy!

The Technology Partners

AI apprised the physician of updated information in the patient's chart before the visit and also sorted out her emails, so her inbox wasn't so full. As well, it automated tasks such as scheduling, billing, and quality control and thus, prevented the physician from wasting time on tasks indirectly related to patient care.

Voice technology not only cut down on the doctor's keyboard clicks for tasks such as retrieving needed information but also saved her the time it would have taken to write visit notes. AI coupled with voice technology listened to the unfolding visit and fashioned the notes.

Other technological advances were similarly helpful in reducing the doctor's workload. Remote monitoring allowed important information about the patient to be instantly sent to the physician. She, in turn, was able to send information immediately to the patient's home. She sent Rhonda the domestic robot new meal plans, exercise plans to the entertainment center, and the pharmacy state-of-the-art earplugs. In addition, the patient's remote monitoring systems at home will monitor his progress and send monthly updates to the physician, who can make adjustments if needed.

Also, since automation decreases in-person visits, it creates less need for office staff, which means less overhead for the practice. In turn, this may eventually yield cheaper co-pays for the patient.

Communication Conundrum: Resolved

While the scenario presented in this chapter may appear to overly idealize the coming impact of technology on healthcare, I believe it's within our grasp. With the assistance of new technology, the communication conundrum can be significantly improved, even resolved, on a number of levels. In Chapter 1, we reviewed the communication categories: societal, institutional, group, interpersonal, and intrapersonal.

With the help of technology, the communication conundrum in this scenario was resolved in multiple ways. On a societal level, an idealized patient-physician bond was more closely realized because both parties had time to discuss the matters which meant the most to them. On an institutional level, the patient-physician bond was a priority—the patient didn't have to take time off work and the physician only had to concentrate on the patient. On a group level, the patient's treatment plan and the physician's workflow were optimized so both parties could spend more time with their families. On an interpersonal level, both the patient and physician were able to communicate their needs and felt listened to by the other party. Finally, on an intrapersonal level, both felt their time was well spent. The patient got the answers he needed, and the physician felt fulfilled by helping her patient.

Treating the Patient Instead of the Disease

In addition to solving the communication conundrum, technology frees up the physician's time and energy, which can then be directed toward nuances affecting patient-physician communication; nuances such as cultural rapport. Professor Andy Molinsky developed a six-dimensional approach to diagnosing cultural differences. It addresses directness, enthusiasm, formality, assertiveness, self-promotion, and personal disclosure.[21] For example, in Germany, communication tends to be extremely direct, whereas in Japan, communication is more indirect. Americans, for example, tend to be more enthusiastic than the British, who are generally more reserved.

Another example of nuance in communications theory is how an event is remembered. In his 2010 TED talk, Daniel Kahneman discussed the concept of the "remembering" self, versus the "experiencing" self. The experiencing self is what we experience in the present moment. The remembering self is made of up recalled stories. For example, if you attend a ballet performance, the experiencing self is viewing, hearing, and sensing the performance. The remembering self is remembering what you experienced in the past, for example your childhood ballet lessons or taking your own children to dance class. Significantly, the remembering self makes choices going forward.[22]

Why is this important in medicine?

If two patients go to a physician because of a hand laceration, both may receive the same quality of care. But toward the end of stitching up the laceration, one patient experiences pain while the other did not. That slight but remembered pain constitutes a negative ending which means this patient is less likely to seek care from this physician again despite receiving the same quality of care.

While most physicians don't have formal training in communication nuances, we have more resources at our disposal than we may realize: we must simply use our gifts as human beings. Physicians, through observing vocal intonation, facial expressions, or speech patterns, can often sense how to improve communication. If technology frees up our energy and time, we have a greater chance of using our senses. Therefore, we have a greater chance of determining whether a patient prefers a direct or indirect manner of conversation, of ending an appointment on a positive note, and of treating the whole patient instead of just the disease state.

SECTION TWO:

THE SPACE BETWEEN

UNIT TWO

Chapter 5: Story. Presence. Engagement.

IN THE X-MEN MOVIE franchise, Professor Charles Xavier is a powerful telepath. He also has a perpetual optimism regarding the ability of people to recover after they stumble.[23] Physicians could use a bit of this optimism when it comes to treating patients.

Despite the best of intentions, patients often don't follow through on treatment plans. The enthusiasm which immediately follows a visit often quickly evaporates. Since it's likely to be a few months before a follow-up visit, much or even most of the advice from the last appointment has to be revisited. Generally, a doctor doesn't mind this happening once but may become frustrated if it keeps occurring. Given that physicians often see themselves as time-starved and resource-poor, they may ration their positive energy and lose hope for patients who continually fail to follow their treatment plans.

In cases like this, technology can play a saving role.

Medicine has three legs: medication, surgery, and lifestyle change. It's this last leg, lifestyle change, which could be exponentially boosted by improving patient education through technology. After all, no matter how effective the patient-physician visit, what's the point if the medical treatment plan isn't enacted between appointments?

How do we enhance patient education?

From 2015 until 2018, as part of my overall quest to better communicate with patients, I explored an unlikely pathway for a doctor: comedy. I spent time learning and actually performing as a comedian.

During this adventure, three communication themes emerged: story, presence, and engagement. I came to the realization, as these lessons percolated within me, that comedic communication strategies, paired with specific technological advances, can improve patient education between clinic visits in multiple ways.

The Power of Story in Medicine

A story is a narrative, either real or fictional. It recounts certain events or people for purposes such as entertainment, information, or inspiration. Story is at the center of a comedian's repertoire. Whether writing a sketch, improvising a scene, or telling a set of jokes around a premise, a comedian is relating a story.

What does a story need in order to be effective with patients?

For any story to succeed, it must be in a language the patient can understand. It has to be jargon-free and conversational in tone. Also, it's beneficial to keep the story short. If a story to help a patient understand medical concept goes on too long, you may lose their attention. Most importantly, the story must educate the patient in a palatable fashion.

How does this apply to patient education?

Essentially, a physician could use this concept of story to put complex health information into language which patients can easily understand, retain, and relate to on a human level. Instead of reading down a list of obscure symptoms and signs, sharing an unfolding story that weaves in aspects of the medical condition will enhance patient understanding.

What does technology have to do with it?

The technology tool of trans-media story-telling has the capability to transform story into an powerful communication tool.

Trans-Media Storytelling

In simple terms, trans-media storytelling is when a story is told across multiple media channels such as movies, video games, and comics. The individual story consumed on one platform may provide a great experience. However, if the combined stories are consumed over all the platforms, the audience has a much richer experience.

An example of trans-media storytelling in the film industry is the "Marvel Universe" of films, which includes many movies based upon comic book heroes such as *Iron Man*, *Spider Man*, *Black Panther*, and *The Avengers*. Many of these characters also appear in other media channels such as comic books, and video games. This means the audience can experience the individual story of a particular fictional hero solely in a movie or get a larger narrative by adding the comic book or video game.[24]

Trans-media Storytelling for Healthcare

Healthcare settings may not have the budgets of blockbuster movie franchises, but technology is getting cheaper. For example, let's say a cardiologist wants to tell the story of how a heart attack can occur. A doctor could use a video set in an office to tell the story of a patient having a heart attack at work. Or a physician could tell the story of recovery in a graphic novel the patient could take home. Such storytelling could include heart attack physiology and pathology in a relatable language. Neither the video nor the novel need to be of Hollywood quality. But for patients at risk of having a heart attack—a common condition seen by cardiologists—this would be a great way to transmit important information on a regular basis.

Well-placed humor can also help story delivery. Of course, the humor has to be in good taste and wide enough in appeal to satisfy most audiences, given the diverse background of patients. When humor is used effectively, it can soften the harsh realities of a medical diagnosis or treatment options.

At the end of the day, storytelling is one of the most powerful ways to present ideas to the world. Trans-media storytelling is even more powerful. Why not use this superpower to educate and benefit patients?

The Power of Presence in Medicine

Presence, in its simplest form, is the act of existing in the present moment. In the world of comedy, one has to be in the present to connect with the audience. Not only do you have to perform your own routine, but you have to really listen to the audience. You can take the exact same routine, perform it at two different times and locations, and have two completely different experiences based on the audiences to which the comedian has to react. To react effectively to each audience the comedian has to be highly aware of the audience and be spontaneously creative.

What sort of presence do physicians need with patients?

For patients to feel as though they are being heard, a physician needs to listen to a patient's words and also to their vocal tone, body language, and facial gestures. If patients sense that their medical provider is truly present and paying attention to them, then they will feel a connection and pay more attention.

How does this apply to patient education?

Even if the doctor explains the patient's medical condition in a relatable story, the power of this story is further enhanced if the patient can feel a connection to the story—especially if they feel that they are a part of the story. They'll be able to transform their medical condition from an abstract concept to an active part of their existence. This may help boost a patient's motivation to change.

What does technology have to do with it?

Technology can intensify the power of presence through altered reality, which can be virtual or augmented. Virtual reality is when a person is immersed in a completely different world. Augmented reality is when facets of a fictional world are superimposed upon the real world.

Virtual Reality

In his nonfiction book called *Future Presence*, Peter Rubin describes a virtual reality situation in which people from all over the country came together in a virtual reality setting through avatars. They became friends and two of the participants even got married.[25] While I am not sure how soon it'll be before online dating websites will incorporate virtual reality into their dating options, many professions are considering the benefit of virtual reality. In 2015, indie author Joanna Penn described the concept of a virtual bookstore, where readers could enjoy virtual experiences with authors.[26]

At one point I tried a virtual reality experience called the "Occulus Rift."[27] Unfortunately, I had motion sickness. This can happen when there is a gap between what your eyes see and your body senses. I seem to have a sensitive system. As technology improves, I'm sure the common complaint of motion sickness will be addressed.

Does virtual reality mimic all the senses? Not quite. It's already good at mimicking sight and sound, and currently there's research underway to mimic touch feedback, which is called "haptic feedback." Once this is accomplished, the immersive experience of virtual reality will be much closer to actual reality. There doesn't seem to be as much work on mimicking taste or smell, as compared to touch. This seems less important to most people.[28]

As a neurologist who has had to complete many brain death exams, it makes sense to me that mimicking touch is important in a virtual environment. After a patient dies, loved ones can invoke sight and sound by looking at photographs or videos. They can invoke scent by smelling an old piece of clothing. Associated taste may be recalled by eating familiar foods. But for the loved one, the sense of touch is permanently gone. With the help of technology, who knows what may happen in the future?

Virtual Reality in Medicine

Virtual medicine is a growing trend in medical settings. Dr. Bertalan Mesko, a medical futurist, has noted a number of virtual reality mechanisms that can benefit medicine.[29]

First of all, it can teach medical students about empathy. For example, a virtual reality headset that mimics a stroke deficit would give students a real-life sensation of the neurological experience for stroke patients.

Virtual reality is also a good place to practice medical skills, from delivering bad news to doing a complex surgery.

Immersing patients in virtual reality worlds can also be a great way to make medical procedures more palatable. For example, a child could be immersed in virtual reality while getting a vaccine.

A psychiatric application of virtual reality has been used to decrease patient phobias. If someone is frightened of heights, for example, one can slowly be exposed to the fearful stimulus without being placed in real danger. However, due to the immersive environment's power to trick the mind, the user really does think that the fearful stimulus is real.

Virtual reality is used to manage or decrease pain associated with giving birth. By focusing on virtual reality, the patient's own sensation of pain may decrease, and in the future, this could cut or reduce the need for painkillers.

Finally, at the end of life, virtual reality could make it easier for patients to let go of unfulfilled desires.[30]

It's also possible to use online virtual communication communities in healthcare settings. In particular, I believe this has great potential to alleviate loneliness in the elderly or the disabled who may not be able to venture out to see their friends and loved ones. Harvard University conducted one of the longest studies on happiness, concluding that the key factor in longevity is human connection.[31]

Loneliness is in effect a silent killer. This is a problem for the elderly as their peer group dies out and illness may affect mobility. Virtual reality could create a book club for elderly people around the world or enable elderly people to enjoy activities they can no longer physically do, such as mountain climbing.[32]

When virtual reality is used in a hospital or clinical setting, the patient can be monitored for symptoms of motion sickness and treated appropriately. However, the motion sickness occurring from home use of virtual reality can be a major hindrance, especially to the elderly or disabled populations which would most benefit from the technology. These at-risk populations tend to have medical conditions, which can be adversely affected by technology-induced motion sickness. These are also the populations least likely to have easy access to help if something were to happen at home. Until the motion sickness can be resolved in this population, use of virtual reality will be limited.

Augmented Reality

Even though augmented reality doesn't get the same great press as virtual reality, its sexier cousin, in many ways it has greater potential. I believe we'll see a higher market penetration of augmented reality before the full-market penetration of virtual reality into medicine. Augmented reality is cheaper because of lower manufacturing costs. In the cash-strapped healthcare industry, this price differential is quite significant.

The mass adoption of augmented reality began in 2016 with the phenomenon of great numbers of Americans (and others around the world) trying to catch Pokemon characters while playing "Pokemon Go." Essentially, people would carry their smartphones around as they walked in their normal environments, looking for virtual characters superimposed on regular streetscapes, homes, trees, and so on.[33]

The concept of augmented reality is no longer limited to select images. Both the University of Washington and Facebook built apps which animate stationary elements in an image. In an otherwise still photo, a person will sprint toward you out of the background, or the flames in a hearth fire suddenly lick and flicker upward."[34] The concept once depicted as fictional in the Harry Potter novels may soon become fact.

Augmented Reality in Medicine

During a visit to a Microsoft store in early 2018, I tried the "Hololens," a holograph computer experience using a virtual headset, which delivers augmented reality.[35] At first, it was a bit distracting to have images superimposed on the real world in front of me. However, I didn't find it as disorientating as virtual reality. It was cool to superimpose images on different objects in the store while discussing the experience with another person. I could imagine this technology in use in the medical office. Wouldn't it be cool if the physician and the patient could put on something like the Hololens? They could see a live example of how a drug works, what happens when a person has a heart attack, or where a body part is located.[36]

Another example of augmented reality is the Autism Glass Project using Google-developed eyeglasses. Autistic children often have difficulty recognizing facial expressions and the emotions they represent. When looking through these glasses, the child sees an array of face icons in an upper corner which illuminate that person's emotions. This has wonderful implications to enable better communication, socialization, and interaction for autistic children.[37]

Why not have similar eyeglasses for physicians, which would provide insights in an upper corner regarding our patient's mood? Is the patient happy or sad about what's happening in the visit? So often, what is said in a visit doesn't reflect what a patient is thinking or feeling. It would be wonderful to know if the information we provide to our patients is truly being well received. Of course, such glasses should only be used with the permission of the patient.

The Power of Engagement in Medicine

Engagement is the manner in which a person is interested in a task, issue, or event. In comedy, if there isn't a strong element of active audience engagement, the performance can go downhill even with a great story and well-grounded presence.

Unless patients are engaged in a medical treatment plan, they won't follow through. The patient has to understand the reasons for the treatment plan. Why should they follow it? What's in it for them? Why does it make things better for them?

How does this apply to patient education?

If we can understand the patients' "why," which is their goal for their experience of life, then we can tailor the education of the treatment plan to match their needs. For example, a physician may want a patient who is about to retire soon to increase exercise. By learning that the patient wants to travel during retirement, the physician can include education on how exercise can improve the travel experience. To keep the patient engaged over the long term in improving his or her health, patient education has to be actively interesting and creative.

What does technology have to do with this?

Games can help optimize patient education, keep that education actively interesting, and boost engagement.

Gamification

Games, from Mahjong in China to Carroms in India, can be traced back thousands of years. While games can keep a person engaged, there is more to gamification than simply translating information into a game.

A game designer uses two major elements to motivate people to achieve their goals: game mechanics and experience design.

Game mechanics include points, reward badges, and leader boards, in which one player is compared to other players in the game. For example, in the video game Tetris, there are points for being able to make lines disappear, and you can compare your score relative to other players in the game.

Experience design includes a focus on the actual journey of the player through the game utilizing the storyline, avatars, roleplay, and setting.

Gamification can help motivate people either by changing behaviors or developing new skills. However, increasing motivation is often more complex than just giving points or reward badges. In his book *Drive,* Daniel Pink argues that the old thinking about motivation, which is based on extrinsic factors of reward systems or punishment fears, is ineffective.[38] Instead, he believes that true human motivation stems from intrinsic factors and that people need autonomy, mastery, and purpose to be motivated. In other words, if a person is self-directed, has the urge to improve, and has the desire for something meaningful, then that person is ready to be motivated. This means that a game capable of triggering internal motivation is going to be more successful than one focussing only on external motivation.

Gamification in The Medical Setting

Medicine already has many examples of game usage. For example, "Remission" is a game in which cancer patients receive incentives to follow through on treatment plans.[39] Perhaps the most impressive application of gamification on a major scale in the world of health was developed by Jane McGonigal, a Stanford game designer who turned complications from a concussion into a popular game called "Superbetter." Every day, Jane would go on a little quest to help her condition. She called herself "Jane the Concussion Slayer." Eventually, thousands of people joined in on the game, and in the process, many improved their conditions.[40]

Why was "Superbetter" so successful? Obviously, part of the fun was picking an avatar and earning rewards for completing quests. In addition, perhaps the camaraderie of other players fighting their own battles had a positive impact.

From my medical perspective, however, the greatest benefit was allowing players to choose their own quests to help their individual situations. I believe that this individualization increases a patient's sense of control and therapeutic investment. Granted, you cannot have people make up every part of a treatment plan. But allowing some choice can go a long way in building a patient's sense that they have a stake in the overall health condition. This choice encourages skill improvement and increases the likelihood that the patient will follow the course of treatment and improve health outcomes. Enabling the patient to be self-directed encourages mastery, inspires purpose, and directly ties into intrinsic motivation.

Deflating the Stigma

One prejudice which arises at the mention of gaming or video gaming is the stereotype of a disaffected youth sitting alone in the living room playing a violent video game that features shooting guns. As a physician, I see the national gun violence epidemic in the United States as a public health crisis. Therefore, taking measures to prevent gun violence is very important to me. However, the assumption that video gaming leads inevitably to gun violence in every player is unfair and not representative of the vast majority of gaming enthusiasts, especially those who use gaming for medical purposes.

People may also worry that excessive gaming is addictive. Recently, the World Health Organization recognized a condition called "gaming disorder" in which people are classified as having a medical condition if gaming interferes with their daily functionality.[41] However, a gaming disorder is like any other addiction, and certainly not everyone who enjoys gaming is addicted to it. For example, people who drink a few glasses of wine with friends over the weekend are unlikely to be alcoholics, but someone who has two or more drinks every night and cannot function at work the next morning has a drinking disorder and needs treatment. It is a continuum. Gaming is no different than any other addiction disorder and needs to be treated as such.

Before slamming the whole concept of gamification, it's important not to shoot down an idea before it has a chance to be developed properly and safely. At its core, gaming has great potential to not only teach patients about their medical conditions but also to spark interest in getting treatment for those medical conditions. Will Wright, the creator of the "Sim City" video game, notes that while movies can give one a sense of empathy, games give the player a sense of agency.[42] I agree that one powerful tool in motivating patients to stay the course with treatment is a sense of agency, or a sense of control. So, don't shut out a perfectly good tool for medical education due to an undue prejudice. Instead, we should utilize gamification, with all of its benefits, in combination with trans-media storytelling and altered reality, to help patients back up when they stumble through treatment, education, and recovery.

Chapter 6: Mr. Scotty Spock 3.0

"It is not faith in technology. It is faith in people."

—*Steve Jobs*

WHILE TECHNOLOGY CONTINUES TO expand, it can be tempting to put all our faith in technology to heal the patient. However, unless people properly use technology, it will not help the patient. In the last chapter, we discussed how the concepts of story, presence and engagement can help improve patient education in between appointments. As we discussed, improving patient education is very important in order to engender positive lifestyle changes, which in turn can enhance patients' health.

In order to exemplify the concept of how story, presence, and engagement can improve patient education and in turn improve a patient's well-being, let's return to Mr. Scotty Spock and his insomnia. We last saw him finishing a successful appointment with Dr. Dianna Crusher. However, he faced three long months before his next clinical appointment. Shortly after that last visit, to increase his chances for overall well-being, Dr. Crusher decided to give him a safety net to ensure proper patient education. She deployed an app to help him.

The Sweet Sleep Escape App

After his last appointment with Dr Crusher, Mr. Scotty Spock was quite happy with the treatment plan. His new earplugs fit snugly and blocked out sound. Following the nutrition plan was easy because Rhonda the robot was making delicious meals. The exercise plan was a joy because he got to spend time with his kids. He was even getting a good night's sleep.

Everything was going well until two weeks after his last doctor's appointment when he was assigned a big project at work. On the one hand, he was glad his boss had so much faith in him. On the other hand, he was stressed out by the new responsibilities. Because his mind was churning at night, once again he had trouble getting to sleep, even with the earplugs. To get his work done, he had begun skipping his playdates with his kids. To top it all off, he had started snacking on junk food at work to relieve his anxiety.

At the start of week three, Scotty's computer gently reminded him that he needs to start exercising and eating well again to ease his insomnia. He looked at the prompt and wondered, "*Exactly what was insomnia again?*" Dr. Crusher had covered the topic in detail, but he had forgotten most of what she'd said. After the appointment, she had given him access to a smartphone app called, "The Sweet Sleep Escape." He had forgotten to use it, but he knew he had slid off his treatment plan. He decided to give the app a try.

Story

Mr. Scotty Spock opens up the app. He first creates an avatar. He chooses to be a look-alike of Captain Jean-Luc Picard, but with neon jet-blue hair. Mr. Spock asks the app, "*What is insomnia?*" Then, after switching to full screen mode, the app begins to roll an animated short-story film of his avatar experiencing insomnia. This funny, short video teaches the basics of what insomnia is, how it works in the brain, and why it is important to modify behaviors to treat it. Mr. Scotty Spock congratulates himself for relearning what insomnia is and understanding the importance of behavioral changes in treating it.

Newly inspired, he returns to exercising by playing with the kids and eating Rhonda's cooking. Once again, for another week, this healthy pattern works well for him.

Presence

Unfortunately, once again his sleep troubles return, even though he is exercising, eating right, and wearing his earplugs at night. What he needs now is to use other aspects of the app: a sensory inventory and the power of presence to examine his sleep environment and determine what other factors may need to be modified.

Scotty really tries to comply with the demands of the sensory inventory. Every morning he tells his smartphone what bothered him or helped him during the night. For example, the streetlight disturbed him, or his new mattress was better but still not firm enough. It's relatively easy to supply helpful details as he talks into his phone and walks around his bedroom. When he holds up the phone to the window and talks about the light coming in from the street, the app suggests blackout curtains, finds online vendors, and offers to order curtains matching the window's dimensions. Or when he points to the mattress, the app does another online search and recommends a firmer mattress or maybe different pillow options. All these options show up in an augmented reality format to help the patient understand how these changes would promote better sleep by making his bedroom more environmentally friendly.

The blackout curtains and firmer mattress help, and Scotty's sleep does improve, but he is frustrated because he still has trouble sleeping through the whole night.

Engagement

What he may need now is motivation to improve his sleep hygiene. I believe Scotty must take advantage of the next feature of our app: the power of engagement.

Once again Scotty begins his morning by opening up the app. The app suggests a number of different quests to help his sleep hygiene. One pathway could be a quest to create a good bedtime ritual, such as meditation, yoga, reading, or listening to stories. There is even a podcast designed to put people to sleep by telling boring stories.[43] Another pathway might be to make the bedroom more appealing to a person's sense of smell by washing the linens more regularly or using an essential oil such as lavender.

Scotty chooses the quest of creating a bedtime ritual. The app then gives him suggestions. He picks the combination of listening to a fiction book, doing deep-breathing exercises, and then listening to relaxing music. He tries this for a week, logging how he feels about the sleep rituals every morning. Soon he sees that he falls asleep well, but only after listening most of the night to his favorite audiobook. Therefore, he alters his sleep ritual. He begins with a stretching regimen, then deep-breathing exercises, and tops it off with relaxing music. He tries this for two weeks and finds that it is successful. Then he selects his next quest of improving mindfulness during the day to help with nighttime sleep.

The beauty of this approach is that Scotty can choose which pathway to follow and at what time. The app will award Scotty achievement medals when he completes quests. Additionally, it provides both Scotty and Dr. Crusher with feedback as to the success of specific gaming experiences, including how long and when each intervention was tried. This is critical information, since often the factors which make the biggest difference in successful treatments for insomnia are not only what is tried, but when and for how long the specific intervention is tried.

Redefining Mr. Scotty Spock

When it's time for his three-month follow-up appointment with Dr. Dianna Crusher, Scotty reports significant improvement in his insomnia. He has optimized his sleep environment and improved his sleep hygiene. (Dr. Crusher already knows this before the appointment, because the app has supplied new data and information for her to review.) Because Scotty is sleeping better, his exercises are more effective, and he has lost some weight. All in all, both doctor and patient are pleased with his progress.

Sweet Sleep Escape App Versus the Office Visit

If I had access to something akin to the Sweet Sleep Escape app with my sleep patients, it would make my clinical practice much richer. First of all, when I discuss insomnia, I normally dive into a boring discussion of the three P's, which define insomnia:

1. Predisposing genetic factors such as being prone to light sleep.
2. Precipitating factors such as noisy traffic outside or noisy upstairs neighbors.
3. Perpetuating factors such as exposure to electronic devices which decrease melatonin secretion.

Then, I go on to describe the "reticular activating system," in which the sleep-wake cycle is less like an electric on and off switch and more like a seesaw, with one side balanced toward sleep and the other side balanced toward wakefulness. To treat insomnia, you have to decrease factors which promote wakefulness and increase factors which increase sleep.

Patient's often frown and find it hard to relate to this discussion. I don't blame them! Instead of this boring description of insomnia, wouldn't it be better to tell the story of someone experiencing insomnia, incorporating medical facts into the story? By creating a simple, funny animated video that tells the patient a story of insomnia, the Sweet Sleep Escape App, delivers the medical facts in a relatable manner. Better yet, by becoming an avatar in the story, this only further enhances the story's message.

In terms of sleep environment modification, this is normally a laborious process in the clinical office. In the treatment of this disease, the sleep environment is a highly critical piece of the puzzle because insomniacs can be very sensitive to environmental stimuli.

To assess possible problems, my normal procedure is to ask patients to complete what I call a "five-sense bedroom inventory." For the first two weeks patients must note any smells that help or hinder their sleep. Then for the next two weeks they do the same with sound. This inventory continues with all the five senses. The inventory helps identify which abnormal environmental stimuli are impacting the patient's senses, which in turn negates their ability to sleep. Then, we suggest environmental changes to improve the patient's sleep environment.

However, in my clinical practice I have discovered that often this sensory inventory is simply too labor-intensive for many patients. In addition, their reporting of environmental issues is inaccurate because they lack the energy or will to complete the inventory. Also, unless the physician is shown a detailed photograph of the bedroom, suggested environmental changes are too loosely based upon general descriptions rather than specific conditions. If the patient could use augmented reality to identify problem areas, the therapeutic process would be greatly accelerated. This is what the Sweet Sleep Escape App accomplished in our patient scenario.

In terms of sleep hygiene behavior, this is also a very intensive process in the clinical office. Before we start the process of correcting sleep hygiene, we need to get an idea of what the patient is willing to modify. If the patient is addicted to nighttime reruns of *Monty Python*, cutting late-night viewings may not be a good first step. However, if a patient suffers with knee pain from an old sports injury, perhaps a stretching ritual before to bed would be welcome. Finding what will work for each individual patient is a constant process of trial and error. Complicating this matter is that the treatment which works on one patient at one point in time may not work for the same patient at a different point in time. Therefore, due to the constant trial and error, it is easy for patients to get discouraged when it comes to correcting sleep hygiene. Yet, with a gamified system such as the Sweet Sleep Escape App, patients can have fun with the treatment plan.

I am confident that self-direction, specifically the patient choosing which game to choose as his or her personal quest, can be even more helpful and yield better treatment outcomes than receiving achievement medals or feeding data back to the physician. Self-direction encourages patients to continue working on lessening insomnia, gives patients a greater understanding of the treatment of their condition, and enhances their purpose of playing the games to treat the insomnia. These intrinsic factors, which are linked to gamification, will have a positive impact on changing behaviors and developing new habits.

Therefore, gaming will help insomnia patients, like Scotty, who struggle with how to maintain the commitment to follow their treatment plans. A few weeks after an office visit, enthusiasm may begin to wane. Life kicks in, and patients get busy with other matters. With gamification's reinforcement, however, even when life kicks in, the patient can stay on the treatment track!

Some Technological Questions Answered

After reading so much theoretical material, you may have some lingering questions:

1. Only one story was told in the animated funny video. Was trans-media storytelling used in the app?

The answer is yes, it was used because the digital platforms of the game and altered reality expand the patient's story into the treatment phase. Multiple digital platforms were employed to add different elements of the story. Hence, it was a trans-media storytelling experience.

2. Why did you include augmented but not virtual reality?

It is true that a virtual reality experience may enhance the storytelling aspect of the app and the treatment options it suggests. It's also true that using simpler tools can reduce the cost of virtual reality (e.g. Google Glasses versus Magic Leap virtual reality systems).

However, as a clinician, I made a choice to omit virtual reality in favor of augmented reality for a few specific reasons:

- Motion sickness: as mentioned in the last chapter, the issue of motion sickness at home would make an insomnia app useless.
- Risk of negative experience: once a patient has a negative experience with a treatment modality, it is very hard to get them to use it again.

- Risk of over-stimulation: depending on the virtual reality experience, it may over-stimulate the patient and actually lessen the ability to sleep. With over-stimulated senses, it is hard to turn off the wake system and go to sleep.

In the future, virtual reality worlds may be tempered to help induce rather than negate sleep. However, without real world testing, I determined it was a safer bet to go with augmented reality for beneficial, mass therapeutic adoption.

3. How does the app track sleep environment changes, deliver usable data to the medical provider, and suggest new quests in the game of improving sleep hygiene?

The answer is AI. While this was not expressly discussed in this specific model, in the future, AI will be the juice that provides the therapeutic benefit of successful patient education models.

4. Why would a patient be motivated to use the Sweet Sleep Escape app when there are already so many digital distractions on top of real-world responsibilities?

It's because the gamification component increases intrinsic motivation, which is a powerful method to activate improved health behaviors.

5. Could such a model work for different medical conditions?

As a sleep physician, I have described a theoretical app for insomnia to demonstrate this technology-enabled patient education model, but I am sure that there are plenty of medical conditions well-suited to such an approach. Examples include weight reduction to decrease coronary risk, or diet modification for gastrointestinal illnesses.

To create an effective therapeutic model, it would take a team made up of technologists and medical specialists: technologists to know what is both possible and economically feasible, and medical specialists who understand what is medically important and medically beneficial.

In summary, trans-media storytelling helps the patient understand the disease state and the path to wellness. Altered reality, whether augmented or virtual, can enhance the presence of the patient within the disease state and offer different treatment options. Gamification helps focus on the patient's "why" in the treatment of the disease state. Finally, all three components can be put together in a model which may use something as simple as a patient's smartphone to educate them about a medical condition and enhance behavioral treatment options between clinic visits.

The real power of this model is not in the technology but the patient's response. Because the patient is more likely to accomplish behavioral change, the physician is more likely to have increased faith in the patient. The patient-physician relationship is therefore strengthened. The beauty of this technology model is its ability to increase faith in people.

Chapter 7: Mr. Scotty Spock 4.0

IN THE PAST, SCIENTIFIC breakthroughs of "today," would take a long time to affect the everyday clinical practice of tomorrow. However, the distance between what is today and will be tomorrow is rapidly decreasing. In the next few decades, we'll see seismic shifts in technology which will affect patients and physicians alike. Therefore, treating patients such as Mr. Scotty Spock will be radically different in many ways.

Let's examine some of these changes.

The Artificial Intelligence Occupational Shift

Whether we like it or not, AI is here to stay. The pace of technological change is only increasing, and we're seeing the potential for whole sectors of occupations to be destroyed.

For many people, a job is more than a source of income, it's also a major source of meaning. It's not uncommon for some people, especially those over forty, to define their lives by their work. So, what are we humans supposed to do when AI takes away our jobs? How are we supposed to define our lives? How are we supposed to differentiate ourselves in the world of AI?

In his April 2018 TED talk, Dr. Kai-Fu Lee noted that AI will replace repetitive jobs like customer support and telephone sales within five years, routine jobs like truck drivers and hematologists in ten years and optimizing jobs such as radiologists and reporters in fifteen years. According to Dr. Lee, this massive disruption will lead to major psychological stress for humanity.[44]

Dr. Lee also identified the jobs where human compassion could be wrapped around AI. For example, the elderly could be helped by intelligent robots but would still benefit from a human elderly care companion. He also cited jobs, such as chief executive officers, that are uniquely human and involve creativity and compassion.

I believe, too, that the rollout of 5G connectivity is a major game-changer for humanity in terms of increased connectivity and the disruption of some occupations. As the fifth generation of wireless networking technology, 5G is supposed to be ten times faster than Google fiber's standard home-broadband services and six hundred times faster than the 4G mobile speed on existing smartphones.[45]

> "From artificial intelligence and self-driving cars to telemedicine and mixed reality as yet undreamt technologies, all the things we hope will make our lives easier, safer and healthier will require high-speed, always-on internet connections."
> — Klint Finley, the Wired Guide to 5G

With 5G connectivity rolling out in limited locations through 2019, and more broadly in 2020, its power to transform our lives will be akin to the introduction of electricity. The increased connectivity will hasten the displacement of individuals doing certain jobs.

The Direct Effect on Healthcare

Within healthcare, technological advances may displace many medical staff. Fewer front-office staff members will be needed for scheduling and check-ins, fewer medical staff will be needed to take vitals, and fewer accounting staff will be needed to send bills. Medical specialties that require minimal patient contact, such as radiology, will most likely also be replaced one day. This cutback in human interactions probably won't matter much to younger patients, say, those under forty, who grew up with technology all around them. Often, when I see the younger generations glued to their phones in my office, I think a little less technology and a little more humanity would be beneficial for them. This concept is especially reinforced by the look of death I get when I tell a teenager to put down the phone and look me in the eyes when talking. Who would have thought that eye contact would become such a revolutionary concept!

However, it's doubtful that the elderly will be as adaptable to this decrease in human interaction. One trend that could help address this is the rise of patient navigators: people who help patients in their journeys through the contemporary healthcare landscape. An important part of a navigator's future duties will likely be helping patients use technology. Yet, more sophisticated technology may be designed with the end user in mind, so in time, the elderly may become more comfortable using it.

The Larger Toll

In terms of the patient-physician relationship, what may matter more than the actual changing of jobs is the effect of these changes on the public's mental health. Medical professionals will likely see a significant increase in mental-health conditions in the next decade.

A changing world order and increased global connectivity will increase peoples' insecurity about their jobs. In his TED talk, Dr. Peter Diamondis estimated that by the end of 2020, five billion of the seven billion people on Earth will be online; an increase of three billion people in just ten years. In addition, China's increasing involvement in AI means the United States will for the first time need to compete for dominance.[46] As well, India, Israel, and many other countries have vibrant technological communities that may also play a major role as the world becomes more integrated.

In addition to the job insecurity from a changing world-order, given that most of the Earth's workforce is going to be displaced by technology over the next few decades, the displaced workforce will need to find a new sense of purpose. This sense of purpose can be created by shifting the energy which was once devoted to the workplace over to new activities such as job training in newly created careers, volunteerism, entrepreneurial pursuits, or other creative endeavors. However, if this shift in previous workplace energy is not successful, the individual may be left without a purpose, which in turn can result in a sensation of displacement and disillusionment.

If the employed worker's insecurity and fears are permitted to fester, or the technology-displaced worker's disillusionment and despair are not addressed, the result will be a population of patients who have negative self-worth. When self-worth is redefined in a negative manner, healthcare providers are likely to see poorer compliance from patients. This is because no matter how far technology advances, a human being is still a human being. As physicians know, patients who do not feel good about themselves are less likely to follow medical advice. This lack of follow-through will have a major impact on the patient-physician relationship.

The Longevity Game

Now and again patients ask me about cryogenics. Given that I'm a neurologist by training, they're interested in my thoughts on preserving oneself over the long term for a future in which one can return. In general, I tend to redirect the question because the real issue is a fear of dying rather than technology. Personally, I have accepted that at some point my loved ones and I will die and never return—that's why time on this earth is so precious. However, we're entering an era in which lives may be greatly extended due to the impact of technology.

In his TED interview with Chris Andersen, Ray Kurzweil discussed the "three bridges" to improved health go hand in hand with technology and life extension.[47] The first bridge is about nutrition and exercise, for instance, technology which helps you eat better. The second bridge is about biotechnology that reprograms genetic processes and thus allows us to overcome disease not only in infants but also in the elderly. An example of this is immunotherapy, which could reprogram our immune systems to kill cancer. The third bridge is about employing nano-technology to improve the immune system and kill all disease, which implies a further and theoretical ability to put an end to the disease-induced death of human beings.

While the concept of the three bridges to life extension is intriguing, Kurzweil has broached an even more revolutionary concept concerning the existence of human-plus-AI. Kurzweil suggests that in the future, we'll be able to extend our minds and create a synthetic neocortex in the cloud: just as a smartphone can connect to the cloud, in the future, our neocortices will also be able to connect to that cloud. In his theory, the non-biological portion of our thinking will live on in the cloud and we'll be able to create technology to lengthen the life of our biological body, or to create backup bodies. Further, given the synthesis of the human neocortex with AI in the cloud, we will expand our intelligence in ways yet to be seen and will create new things that will be understood only by the new synthesis of human and machine. He believes that a large part of this may be possible as soon as 2045.

While these predictions are fascinating, I'm not sure they'll all come to pass. In terms of the three bridges of life extension, the idea that we could not only treat disease, but defeat disease is a wonderful concept. It is one thing to live a long time, but to do so with quality of life is most certainly better than decrepitude. It would be of great benefit to both healthcare providers and patients. However, in reality our medical system is so heavily regulated and slow to adapt that I wonder how fast these bridges of life-extension could fully penetrate our healthcare system.

A key factor is also cost, which is already skyrocketing in the United States healthcare system. Unless the price of future technology is significantly lowered, it will be a long time before mass adoption is possible. However, even in a minimal form, we are likely to see the continued extension of healthier individuals with much longer lifespans than our parents. At a fundamental level this will impact the patient-physician relationship.

Furthermore, the synthesis of humans and AI would generate a host of new treatment challenges for the healthcare provider. How do you treat a creature which is part human and part machine? What about data security? It is one thing to protect the privacy of medical records as we do now, but how about the privacy of our actual brains if they were to be stored in the cloud? Also, what would be the ethics surrounding backup bodies? How many do we get? Can we select a different body each time? How about a body that optimizes the ability to rock climb for a few decades and then later a body that optimizes the ability to dance the tango?

All this being said, I do not think my generation of physicians or even the next generation have to worry about these questions on a mass scale. The technological ability to extend human brains with AI may be present by 2045, but adoption and implementation of such technology will likely be met with great resistance by the mass patient population. No matter what technology can achieve, it must be balanced with the practicality of implementation if it is to affect the patient-physician bond on a large scale.

Technology's Mind Readers

In her TED talk, Nita Farahany discussed the concept of technology being able to read our minds.[48] Currently, in government-run factories in China, workers are forced to wear portable electro-encephalograms to monitor their productivity. Workers can even be sent home if they appear to be distracted. Who is going to help people protect the privacy of their brains? If brains become too transparent, could they be spied upon by governments or could the information be sold by companies to third-party interests? Could people be persecuted for their religious beliefs or political opinions before they are ready to share them publicly? What are we to do to prevent our brains from being hacked and tracked?

I agree with Ms. Farahany. We need to seek better ways to control how our information is given out and legal remedies in case our information is misused. We need to protect our right to cognitive liberty, in which we can think and determine our own futures, including the right to consent to or refuse any type of mind alteration. Cognitive liberty should be a universal human right.

Even though the idea of using technology for brain reading seems far in the future, this may be closer than most people realize, given the rate of exponential increase in technological information. I strongly support protecting our personal cognitive thoughts and emotions against any person, company, or government who could use them to change our inner lives. We need to avoid a scenario such as that in *Minority Report*, in which people are arrested for their thoughts.[49]

On the flip side of the privacy debate, others have noted that humans may actually behave better because their lives are more exposed and that also, when everyone has a more public profile in the future, there may be a lower threshold for privacy—and this will be universally accepted. In some respects, it is true that the threshold for privacy is already lower than it used to be. My younger physician peers are more likely to have public social media accounts with pictures of their loved ones. My generation of physicians tends to be more private in our social media account settings (if we have those accounts at all). In the past, most physicians valued their privacy highly due to their desire to retain a separation between work and home. There is also the fact that, now and again, most physicians have to deal with crazy patients.

The one area of privacy which does concern me greatly is the selling of personal information to third-party sites. Even though the Chinese reveal a great deal more personal data in their technological databases, it is actually illegal in China to sell a person's personal information to a third party.[50] I wish there were such a law in the United States.

The concept of security also goes hand-in-hand with that of privacy. One can have all the privacy measures in the world, but what is the point if the data is hacked? In 2018, Facebook was publicly criticized for selling its user information to Cambridge Analytica, a British political consulting firm which in turn appears to have been used for interference by Russians.[51] In addition, the US government charged China with breaching security, on multiple fronts, for corporate espionage.[52] While it is good that these major breaches received public attention, I also wonder how much more goes on that is not in the realm of public knowledge.

The concept of privacy is even more important in medicine. In the medical setting, it is very important that patients continue to have the freedom to be able to divulge their innermost thoughts and feelings so they can be appropriately treated. Currently, as physicians, we play detective by using what our patients tell and show us through their behavior. What would happen if we could read our patients' thoughts and emotions? A wonderful concept in some respects, but it would have to be done with the explicit permission of the patient. In addition, this information would have to be guarded with the utmost privacy so that it could not be used for other purposes. We need to proceed cautiously so that any such information would be used in a beneficial, transparent manner. Could we guarantee the security of such a healthcare record? A patient's brain data should not be handed or sold to any third party.

No matter what scientific breakthroughs of today lead to in terms of the technology of tomorrow, the implementation of such technology should be guided by the principles of honorable humanity. These core principles are timeless in importance.

Conclusion: Humanity 2.0

> *"A fit body, a calm mind, a house full of love. These things cannot be bought. They must be earned."*
>
> *—Naval Ravikant*

I'D LIKE TO AMEND this intriguing quote slightly, so it applies to the well-being of a patient, to "a heart and house full of love." A patient needs to have a fit body to enjoy life. A patient needs to have a calm mind to experience life. And a patient needs a loving heart and a house of loved ones to savor life.

None of these attributes can be bought on the street. Each has to be earned. A fit body is earned by taking care of oneself through activities such as proper exercise and nutrition. A calm mind is achieved by daily practices such as mindful meditation. A heart and a house full of love are gained by making meaningful connections with other humans and taking the time to fill one's own well with joy. Regardless of how much medicine advances, I believe that if patients can achieve these attributes, they will live a quality life. A strong, communicative patient-physician relationship will further this goal.

In this book, we've covered how the promise of technology can transform patient-physician communication before, during, and after a clinical visit. We've walked through a proposed model to address the problem of patient education between clinical visits. This improved patient-education model serves to further strengthen the patient-physician communication bond. Finally, we discussed the potential impact of future technological transformations on the patient-physician relationship.

I believe that many in healthcare fear technological progress and feel technology will impede rather than help a patient's welfare. Are they right to be fearful? Whether technology will harm or help patients is not really a technological question, but a human one. For example, a drone can be used to deliver medications to a person living on a remote farm or to drop a bomb on a city. Both use the same technology, but its purpose and deployment are determined by the human choice.

In a similar way, technology can be used in healthcare in a manner which benefits all parties, so long as the humans involved choose wisely. I would argue that as technology progresses, the human element will become even more important. Technology cannot mimic human compassion. The healthcare system stands to reap benefits when human compassion is coupled with technological advances.

Otto Knoke, who is sometimes affectionately known as Guatemala's oldest nerd, has used technology to continue his work as a data analyst even after developing Amyotrophic Lateral Sclerosis (ALS). As the paralytic disease progressed, he refashioned a computer mouse as a foot pedal and learned to use eye-tracking software to type.[53]

This capacity to enrich technology with compassion is possible for companies as well as individuals. In 2015, Jini Kim, the founder of a San Francisco start-up called Nuna, developed Medicaid's first centralized and cloud-based data warehouse system. Her motivation stemmed from her youth, when she helped her family get on Medicare so that they would not be burdened by debt resulting from medical bills related to her brother's autism.[54]

Additionally, the technology-plus-compassion equation is well-equipped to ameliorate disease states such as dementia. For example, home sensors can monitor for a patient's wanderings, as well as circadian rhythm patterns. If these assistive technologies are deployed in a manner which can compassionately help, and not hinder the caregiver and health-care provider, they can provide quality care for the vulnerable, dementia population.[55]

Furthermore, the technology-plus-compassion formula has the power to bring about societal change. In her TED speech, American social activist, Ruby Sales noted that technology can provide a larger vista for interaction in which we can learn about each other beyond one's "whiteness, browness or blackness." Technology could be used as a platform to unite instead of segregating people across America, which in turn could strengthen our democracy.[56]

But, how do we leverage compassionate technology on a practical level?

I believe that a framework for action is the key to using the technology-plus-compassion partnership for the greater good of humanity. One such framework is the *Objectives and Key Results (OKR)* framework developed by Andrew Grove, the former CEO of Intel. OKR helps organizations implement strategy through a goal-management framework. Identifying common objectives and up to five key results for employees and their work improves focus and transparency. OKR is used by Bill Gates in Microsoft and the Bill and Melinda Gates Foundation, by rock star Bono and his One charity, which seeks to end global poverty and access to HIV treatment for all, and by others at Google, Zynga, and LinkedIn.[57]

Whatever framework one chooses, what matters is that all the players in the synergy of technology and medicine must have the ability to apply technology for more than the simple metrics of quarterly expense reports, supply-chain statistics, or patient satisfaction scores. Instead, we need to cast the human superpower of compassion onto data metrics. If we combine compassion with accountability, we will have the ability to bring back the beauty in the patient-physician relationship by using technology for humanity's sake rather than for technology's sake. In this manner, we can achieve a wonderful Humanity 2.0, with a fit body, calm mind, and a heart and house full of love.

Appendix

Top Sixteen Resources for the Busy Healthcare Practitioner

If you're interested in reading more about technology and the way in which it will shape the future of healthcare, here are some resources I found useful:

1. **The Medical Futurist:** A blog site, run by Dr. Bertalan Mesko, that also hosts regular YouTube videos. It targets the intersection of healthcare and technology. This is my top resource pick for the busy physician who wishes to stay up-to-date in healthcare technology. The articles and videos are easily digested and as such ideal for the busy practitioner. https://medicalfuturist.com
2. **The Creative Confidence Series Podcast:** This podcast has discussions on leadership and design-thinking. Although it is not actually a technology resource, the humanization of technology is key for healthcare, and design thinking has a key role in this process. Run by IDEO-U. https://www.ideou.com/pages/podcast
3. **Wired:** This journalistic website delivers substantive

information on technology and the intersection of technology and culture.https://www.wired.com

4. **Clear & Vivid:** If you want to learn about communication skills which will benefit the medical provider, this is an excellent podcast which discusses the worlds of communicating and relating. It is hosted by the talented acting-legend Alan Alda. In fact, it is his work on how improvization empowers scientific communication which started me down my quest of comedy, communication and technology. https://www.aldacommunicationtraining.com/podcasts

5. The Wall Street Journal, **"The Future of Everything":** This weekly podcast gives highlights from the world of technology in under thirty minutes. It's a great resource on general trends within technology. https://www.wsj.com/podcasts/wsj-the-future-of-everything

6. **TED Talks Technology:** As you have no doubt already guessed, I am quite a fan of TED talks. Accessible and informative sessions delivered by accomplished leaders in all fields. https://www.ted.com/talks

7. **The Exponential Wisdom Podcast**: A podcast by Peter Diamondis, a thoughtful leader in technology. Each month, often under thirty minutes, the busy practitioner can get a high-level overview of changes in technology. https://www.diamandis.com/podcast

8. **UNSW Trans-Media Storytelling:** One of my next books is on story-telling and medical communication, including trans-media storytelling. For more on this concept, have a look at what's posted by the University of New South Wales in Sydney, Australia, including a recommended introduction to trans-

media storytelling. https://student.unsw.edu.au/ mooc-transmedia-storytelling-narrative-worlds-emerging-technologies-and-global-audiences

9. **SuperBetter:** I briefly discussed this website already, but it gives practitioners a good idea of how gaming can help improve the lives of patients. https://www. superbetter.com

10. **TechAsia:** Technological advances are coming fast and furious from Bangalore, Beijing, and Seoul. https://www.techinasia.com

11. **Stanford Technology Ventures Program:** These Silicon Valley sites may interest health practitioners who want to develop their own start-up or technological advancements. Stanford has long produced technological powerhouses. If you are considering a start-up, Paul Graham's blog is also a good place to begin. He is the founder of the Y-Combinator accelerator for start-ups. https:// sentest.stanford.edu/member/stanford-technology-ventures-program and also http://www.paulgraham. com

12. **Hidden Brain:** This is a podcast from National Public Radio, which discusses the scientific under-pinnings of human behavior. As noted in this book, understanding the human side is key to developing technology which is beneficial to health-care. https:// www.npr.org/podcasts/510308/hidden-brain

13. **Elements of AI:** If you want a free online, quality course on the basics of AI without the need to program, this is a good course from the University of Helsinki. https://www.elementsofai.com

14. **The Grumpy Old Geeks Podcast:** This is a podcast which highlights recent developments in the

world of technology. It is an irreverent podcast and not for those who are offended by swearing, strong language or are sensitive to raw humour. https://www.gog.show

15. **Ready Player One:** (One Bonus Movie Recommendation.) If you are wondering what the world of virtual reality may be like in the future, this is a good movie to enjoy on a weekend evening with some popcorn or milk duds. https://www.imdb.com/title/tt1677720

16. **Star Talk:** (One Bonus Podcast Recommendation.) This is a podcast which combines the worlds of science and pop culture. It is lead by a brilliant, charismatic astro-physicist called Neil deGrasse Tyson. https://www.startalkradio.net

Acknowledgments

It is impossible to thank everybody who inspired me along my author journey. Many people I met briefly, and may not have remembered your name. Please forgive me. Your help was invaluable.

Great thanks to the team who put this book together. I appreciate all that you have taught me Boni, John, and the rest of the team at Ingenium Books.

Enormous thanks to my comedy and design-thinking comrades. I appreciate your teachings Victoria, Suzie and Vidhika, Jay, Derek, Nathaniel, Mathina and Tim.

Eternal gratitude to all the friends and family who urged me onward throughout the years along my author journey. Special thanks to Mahesh, Sowmya, Mani, Praveen, Raja, Pradeep, Thanhvan, Karen, Heidi, Margaret, Tam-Chinh, Laura, Stewie, Kylan, Tina, Aimee, Swathi, Priya and Ellen.

Most of all, a boundless gratitude and thank you to mom and dad. Without both of you I'm nothing!

If you have read this far, I thank you, dear reader, for the gift of your time

About the Author

Pranathi Kondapaneni is a physician, writer and explorer-in-chief. At the age of sixteen, she was accepted into medical school through a combined BA/MD program. By twenty-four, she had completed four degrees in seven years: two bachelor of arts degrees (economics and biology), a master's in public health, and a medical degree. After completing a residency in neurology and two fellowships, one in sleep and the other in epilepsy, Dr. Kondapaneni spent a decade as a private practice attending physician.

Due to her frustration with clinical medicine, Dr. Kondapaneni set out on a series of adventures to help improve communication in the medical office and to combat physician burn-out. These adventures included everything from comedy routines to classes on artistic visual observation. Dr. Kondapaneni enjoys exploring other disciplines in order to find ways to empower physicians to improve communication and combat burn-out.

She lives in Michigan, USA, but has traveled extensively throughout the United States. She's also traveled to Australia, India, Chile, and South Africa. She enjoys listening to audiobooks and podcasts, drinking a good cup of tea, and soaking up culture through art, architecture, food, or a great movie.

Connect with Pranathi and discover more of her work at www.thephysicianphoenix.com.

Endnotes

1   Nadjia Yousif, "Why You Should Treat the Tech You Use at Work Like a Colleague," filmed October 2018 at TED@BCG, TEDx, Toronto, Ontario, Canada, video posted December 2018, https://www.ted.com/speakers/nadjia_yousif.

2   "Hippocratic Oath," Wikipedia, last modified January 5, 2019, https://en.wikipedia.org/wiki/Hippocratic_Oath.

3   Star Trek: The Next Generation, created by Gene Roddenberry, TV series 1987-1994, accessed IMDb January 8, 2019, https://www.imdb.com/title/tt0092455.

4   Coursera, "Introduction to Communication Science," online course offered by the University of Amsterdam, accessed January 8, 2019, https://www.coursera.org/learn/communication

5   Norman Rockwell, Country Doctor, 1947, accessed January 8, 2019, https://prints.nrm.org/detail/260987/rockwell-visiting-the-family-doctor.

6   Norman Rockwell, Country Doctor, 1947, accessed January 8, 2019, https://prints.nrm.org/detail/260987/rockwell-visiting-the-family-doctor.

7   The Nest Home System, accessed January 8, 2019, https://nest.com.

8   Angela Chen, "Why the New Apple Watch with EKG Matters," The Verge, September 12, 2018, https://www.theverge.com/2018/9/12/17850660/apple-watch-series-4-ekg-electrocardiogram-health-2018.

9   "Digital Tattoos Make Healthcare More Visible," The Medical
    Futurist, September 4, 2018, https://medicalfuturist.com/digi-
    tal-tattoos-make-healthcare-more-invisible.

10 Dynamic Body Technology, accessed January 8, 2019, https://
    dynamicbodytechnology.com.

11 "Microsoft Build 2018," conference, filmed May 2018 in
    Seattle, Washington, video, accessed June 2018, https://www.
    microsoft.com/en-us/build.

12 Jillian D'Onifor, Christia Farr, "Google is Hiring People to Work
    on Improving Visits to the Doctor's Office with Voice and Touch
    Tech," CNBC, June 14, 2018, https://sg.finance.yahoo.com/
    news/google-hiring-people-improving-visits-140600223.html.

13 "Iron Man 3," Marvel Studios Movie Released May 3rd, 2013,
    IMDb. Accessed January 8th, 2019. https://www.imdb.com/
    title/tt1300854/

14 Kai-Fu Lee, Artificial Intelligence Superpowers, China, Sili-
    con Valley and the New World Order, performed by Mikael
    Naramore, ch. 1-4, Grand Haven, Michigan, Brilliance Audio,
    audio book, 2018, https://aisuperpowers.com.

15 Kai-Fu Lee, Artificial Intelligence Superpowers

16 Peter Diamandis, AI Superpowers by Kai Fu Lee, tech blog,
    September 4, 2018, https://www.diamandis.com/blog/kai-fu-
    lee-ai-superpowers.

17 Amazon Go, accessed January 8, 2019, https://www.amazon.
    com/b?ie=UTF8&node=16008589011.

18 Waymo, accessed January 8, 2019, https://waymo.com.

19 "Deepmind and Moorfields Eye Hospital NHS Foundation
    Trust," DeepMind, accessed January 8, 2019, https://deepmind.
    com/applied/deepmind-health/working-partners/health-re-
    search-tomorrow/moorfields-eye-hospital-nhs-foundation-trust/.

20   Chris Waugh, "How Design Can Make Healthcare More Human," interview by Suzanne Gibbs Howard, Creative Confidence Series, podcast, December 18, 2018, https://www.ideou.com/blogs/inspiration/how-design-can-make-healthcare-more-human.

21   Andy Molinsky, "How to Extend Reach of Rapport Across Cultures," interview by Jordan Harbinger, The Jordan Harbinger Show, podcast, episode 132, December 10, 2018, https://www.jordanharbinger.com/andy-molinsky-how-to-extend-the-reach-of-rapport-across-cultures.

22   Daniel Kahneman, The Riddle of Experience Vs. Memory, filmed February 2010 at TED2010, Long Beach, California, video, posted March 2010, https://www.ted.com/speakers/daniel_kahneman.

23   X-Men First Class, directed by Matthew Vaughn, Marvel Studios, June 3, 2011, accessed January 8, 2019, https://www.imdb.com/title/tt1270798.

24   "Marvel Cinematic Universe," Wikipedia, last modified January 8, 2019, https://en.wikipedia.org/wiki/Marvel_Cinematic_Universe.

25   Peter Rubin, Future Presence, How Virtual Reality Is Changing Human Connection, Intimacy and The Limits of Ordinary Life, read by Roger Wayne, chapter 7, New York, New York, Harper Collins Publishers, audio book, April 17, 2018, ptr-rbn.com/book.

26   Joanna Penn, "Virtual Reality and the Future of Publishing," The Bookseller, March 16, 2015, https://www.thebookseller.com/futurebook/joanna-penn-virtual-reality-and-future-publishing.

27   "Oculus Rift," Rift, accessed January 8, 2019, https://www.oculus.com/rift.

28 "How Does Medical Virtual Reality Make Healthcare More Pleasant?" The Medical Futurist, April 24, 2018, https://medicalfuturist.com/how-does-medical-virtual-reality-make-healthcare-more-pleasant.

29 How Does Medical Virtual Reality Make Healthcare More Pleasant?

30 How Does Medical Virtual Reality Make Healthcare More Pleasant?

31 Robert Waldinger, What Makes A Good Life? Lessons from The Longest Study on Happiness, filmed November 2015 at TEDx Brookline, MA, December 2015, https://www.ted.com/speakers/robert_waldinger.

32 "The Digital Pickwick Club: A Nursing Home of The Future," The Medical Futurist, September 16, 2018, https://medicalfuturist.com/the-digital-pickwick-club-a-nursing-home-of-the-future.

33 Pokemon Go, accessed January 8, 2019, https://www.pokemongo.com/en-us.

34 Luke Dormehl, "Magical New AR Demo Transforms 2D Photos into Harry Potter-Style 3D Animations," Digital Trends, December 24, 2018, www.digitaltrends.com.

35 "Hololens," Microsoft, accessed January 8, 2019, https://www.microsoft.com/en-us/hololens.

36 Sarah Toy, "Augmented Reality Gives Brain Surgeons A Better View," Healthcare Technology, The Wall Street Journal, May 29, 2018, R2.

37 Autism Glass Project, accessed January 8, 2019, autismglass.stanford.edu.

38 Daniel Pink, Drive: The Surprising Truth About What Motivates Us, narrated by Daniel Pink, audio book, ch 1-4, New

York, New York, Penguin Random House, January 2010, https://www.danpink.com/drive.

39 Pamela M. Kato, Steve W. Cole, Andrew S. Bralyn, Brad H. Polock, "A Video Game Improves Behavioral Outcomes in Adolescents and Young Adults with Cancer. A Randomized Trial," Pediatrics, vol. 122, issue 2, (August 2008).

40 Jane McGonigal, "Superbetter: The Power of Living Gamefully," narrated by Jane McGonigal, audio book, New York, Penguin Audio, ch 1-12, September 15, 2015, https://www.superbetter.com.

41 "World Health Organization Gaming Disorder Classification," World Health Organization, accessed January 8, 2019, https://www.who.int/features/qa/gaming-disorder/en.

42 Will Wright, "Will Wright Teaches Game Design and Theory," masterclass, accessed January 8, 2019, https://www.masterclass.com/classes/will-wright-teaches-game-design-and-theory.

43 Sleep With Me Podcast, accessed January 8, 2019, https://www.sleepwithmepodcast.com.

44 Kai-Fu Lee, How AI Can Save Our Humanity, video filmed April 2018 at TED2018, Vancouver, British Columbia, Canada, August 2018, https://www.ted.com/talks/kai_fu_lee_how_ai_can_save_our_humanity.

45 Klint Finely, "The Wired Guide to 5G," Wired, December 13, 2018, https://www.wired.com/story/wired-guide-5g.

46 Peter Diamondis, Abundance Is Our Future, filmed February 2012, at TED2012, Long Beach, California, video, March 2012, https://www.ted.com/talks/peter_diamandis_abundance_is_our_future.

47 Ray Kurweil, "On What the Future Holds Next," interview by Chris Anderson, The TED Interview, podcast, December 4, 2018, https://www.ted.com/talks/the_ted_interview_ray_kurzweil_on_what_the_future_holds_next.

48   Nita Farahany, When Technology Can Read Minds How Will We Protect Our Privacy, video filmed at TED Salon, Zebra Technologies, New York, New York, November 2018, https://www.ted.com/talks/nita_farahany_when_technology_can_read_minds_how_will_we_protect_our_privacy.

49   Minority Report, directed by Steven Spielberg, June 21, 2002, accessed IMDb January 8, 2019, https://www.imdb.com/title/tt0181689.

50   Dr. Kai-Fu Lee, "AI Superpowers," Abundance Digital Community Webinar, August 2018, accessed December 2018, https://www.diamandis.com/abundance-digital.

51   Nicholas Thompson, Fred Vogelstein, "A Hurricane Flattens Facebook," Wired, March 30, 2018, https://www.wired.com/story/facebook-cambridge-analytica-response.

52   Brian Barrett, "How China's APT10 Hackers Stole the World's Secrets," Wired, December 20, 2018, https://www.wired.com/story/doj-indictment-chinese-hackers-apt10.

53   "Oldest Nerd of Guatemala Types with His Eyes to Modernize Industries," Microsoft YouTube video, September 10, 2018, https://www.youtube.com/watch?v=ZTxjdFJmgwo.

54   Nuna, accessed January 8th, 2019, https://www.nuna.com.

55   Shirley S. Wang, "For Those with Dementia, an Assist from Technology," Healthcare Technology, The Wall Street Journal, May 29, 2018, R8, https://www.wsj.com/articles/for-those-with-dementia-help-from-technology-1527559380

56   Ruby Sales, "How We Can Start to Heal the Pain of Racial Division," video filmed September 2018 at Ted Salon, Verizon, New York, New York, February 1, 2019, https://player.fm/series/tedtalks-audio/how-we-can-start-to-heal-the-pain-of-racial-division-ruby-sales

57 Sarah Berger, "How Bill Gates, Richard Branson and Ray Dalio Approach Goal-Setting," CNBC Make It, January 2, 2019, https://www.cnbc.com/2018/12/27/how-bill-gates-richard-branson-and-ray-dalio-approach-goal-setting--.html?&q-searchterm=THIS%20GOAL%20SETTING%20METH-OD%20IS%20USED%20BY%20BILL%20GATES

www.ingramcontent.com/pod-product-compliance
Lightning Source LLC
LaVergne TN
LVHW092339060326
832902LV00008B/732